THE GOLDEN AGE OF ORTHODONTICS: DECLINE AND AFTERMATH

A History of the Business of Orthodontics

by
Norman Wahl, DDS, MS, MA

The Golden Age of Orthodontics: Decline and Aftermath
Copyright ©2017 Norman Wahl

ISBN 978-1506-904-69-6 PRINT

LCCN 2017948997

September 2017

Published and Distributed by
First Edition Design Publishing, Inc.
P.O. Box 20217, Sarasota, FL 34276-3217
www.firsteditiondesignpublishing.com

To my teachers

Foreword

Dr Norman Wahl's life in our specialty spans much of the era of modern orthodontics. His education included the United States Military Academy at West Point, the University of Illinois College of Dentistry, and the Northwestern University Department of Orthodontics under Chairman Dr John R. Thompson, Drs Hal Perry, Shelly Rosenstein, Todd Dewel, and Harry Sicher. Dr Allan G. Brodie rounded out the list of classic influences. I first met Norm when I was on the Board of Directors of the Pacific Coast Society of Orthodontists (PCSO). He was working on the history of the PCSO and as President I supported his efforts, realizing he was a unique individual with a keen sense of the importance of our history and the literacy skills to make it come to life. As Chairman of the Orthodontic Department at UCLA, I recruited Norm to create and implement a course on orthodontic history for our residents.

His published articles have appeared in many journals including the *PCSO Bulletin, The American Journal of Orthodontics and Dentofacial Orthopedics, The Angle Orthodontist, The World Journal of Orthodontics*, and the *Journal of Clinical Orthodontics*. He has become one of the premier historians in our specialty.

Maybe my fascination with Norm's book is the fact that I've witnessed a lot of what he so eloquently describes. In the mid-1970s, when I started my orthodontic training, our first patients were fully banded (not bonded), most had the extraction of four premolars, and all Class II patients received a headgear. When I finished my training, several of my teachers who invited me to practice with them had waiting lists for patients to start treatment. But fueled by numerous factors that Norm describes, our specialty began to change and change rapidly. And with increasing innovations in treatment methods, technology, business principles, and marketing, our specialty continues to evolve to meet the demands of sophisticated consumers.

The first part of the book, the work primarily associated with Norm's master's thesis in history from California State University at Northridge, can be described as historical. Part II continues the history, but the book takes on a tutorial tone on how to practice in today's competitive, transparent, consumer-oriented, and litigious society.

The knowledge about our specialty that Norm has acquired and methodically outlines in his book is now available to all. It should be required reading for all residents and any orthodontist who wants to know where we've been and where we might be going. As orthodontists we have a noble legacy. I used to tell my students that they were direct descendants (orthodontically speaking) from Dr Edward H. Angle, the father of modern orthodontics. One of my teachers at the University of Washington was Dr Alton W. Moore, founding chair of the department. Al had been trained by

Allan Brodie at the University of Illinois, and Brodie had been trained by Angle. That would make me Angle's grandson—orthodontically speaking—and my students his great-great grandchildren. As Theodore Roosevelt once said, "The more you know about the past, the better prepared you are for the future."

Any accurate historical record will have its unflattering aspects, to say the least. Norm pulls no punches in his assessment of the decline of the golden age of orthodontics and its aftermath. Once I started reading this book, I couldn't put it down. It has been almost 50 years since Norm's first book was published. The wait has been well worth it.

Patrick K. Turley D.D.S., M.S.D., M.Ed.
Professor Emeritus
Section of Orthodontics, School of Dentistry
University of California at Los Angeles

ACKNOWLEDGMENTS

I am deeply grateful to the following individuals for their help and encouragement (1) in writing the thesis: Paul Koistinen, PhD (my graduate advisor); Milton B. Asbell, DDS (now deceased); Jay W. Friedman, DDS; Richard A. Mays, DDS; William S. Parker, DDS (now deceased); and Julian Singer, DDS; (2) in writing the book: Henry D. Hulan; Patrick K. Turley, DDS; David L. Turpin, DDS; Larry W. White, DDS; and (3) for reading both the thesis and the book: Gerald A. Ullman, DDS. To Dr Turley I offer special thanks for going above and beyond the call of duty in his counsel. My gratitude goes to Andrea Matlak of the American Dental Association Library for checking the references. Thanks to my granddaughter, Autumn Rose Wahl, for being my "cover girl." And to my wife, Betty, for all the quality time you gave up so that this book could be realized.

PREFACE

Every field of endeavor—art, music, literature—has its golden age. By this is usually meant the time of greatest achievement, of artistic excellence. The term, "golden age," can also apply to a period of economic plenty for the practitioners of a field such as medicine, law, or architecture.

During the population explosion in the United States following World War II, no group prospered more than orthodontists (relative to its past) because these specialists thrive on a continual supply of young patients. So the period roughly between 1950 and 1970, when the specialty had abundant referrals and a minimum of outside interferences, might be called the golden age of orthodontics.

Before the second war and the Great Depression, there were other periods when orthodontists enjoyed relative security, so it might be argued that these could also be called golden ages. During those years, however, the specialty did not enjoy widespread public acceptance, nor were practitioners' techniques and clinical training so highly developed as they were later.

During the 1960s, health care recipients were becoming more and more aware of certain inequities, especially within the context of the Great Society: Physicians and dentists were poorly distributed, the cost of health care was rising faster than other segments of the economy, health care practitioners enjoyed a disproportionate level of income relative to the general population, and many people could not even get care.

Thus, even before the golden age had peaked, these and other forces began to make themselves felt. They came from many directions: demographic, political, legal, social, economic—even technological advances brought unexpected liabilities.

Two of these forces were especially significant. The first was the marked drop in the number of teenagers—a result of the end of the postwar baby boom. Unlike other health specialists, the orthodontist usually treats a given patient but once, then must seek fresh patients to sustain his or her practice. The second force was a decrease in the busyness of general practitioners (GPs), with the effect that more nonorthodontists were placing braces. For the first time in history, orthodontists found it necessary to cultivate and nurture patient referral sources, and the term "marketing" entered the vocabulary of a staid profession.

Other than reducing the output of new orthodontists (which was only done belatedly and to a limited extent), there was little control the specialty could have exerted in offsetting the effects of a declining patient pool. Concerted action against these forces was overcome by member complacency and (in the case of nonspecialist competition) ruled out by prohibitions against restraint of trade. While the opening of clinics by large corporations was generally decried, these facilities created employment opportunities for many new graduates.

Of course, many of these forces, such as managed care, affected the entire health care industry. What these forces were, how they impacted the specialty, and what efforts were made to deal with them, comprise the core of PART ONE, which was originally a thesis written to partially fulfill the requirement for a master's degree in history at California State University, Northridge, in 1994.

Upon completion of the thesis, my advisors urged me to have it published. However, I made no serious effort to do so until about 17 years later, by which time it would seem that an update was in order. Therefore, I decided to use the thesis as PART ONE and add a PART TWO to cover the period 1997 to the present. However, I thought it might be useful to include, in addition to history, a "how-to" for orthodontists coping with the problems of practicing in the early years of the 21st century.

I began practicing orthodontics in Southern California in 1963, during the waning years of the golden age. Therefore, much of the narrative is based upon firsthand knowledge. Also, California will be mentioned frequently not only because it is the area most familiar to the author, but because it has a high concentration of orthodontists and a reputation for innovation.

We will begin with a brief history of organized orthodontics. As the chronology progresses, less emphasis will be placed on scientific advances and more on the economic and social aspects of the specialty. Although it is assumed that learned men have usually inhabited the upper strata of society, little has been recorded of their economic rank until recent times.

One might ask, "Who cares about a bunch of "fat cats"? Certainly their woes were not on the same level as the poverty, persecution, or famine that other groups had suffered at various times, but in terms of economic history, there may be lessons to learn. Was this group of professionals too self-satisfied? Did they bring misfortune on themselves? Or was the decline inevitable? In retrospect, the golden age of orthodontics may have been just a fortuitous time in the profession's history that was finally brought into step with reality.

Norman Wahl

CONTENTS

LIST OF TABLES

PART ONE

NINETEENTH AND TWENTIETH CENTURIES

CHAPTER I

Early History of Organized Orthodontics

Before the end of the 19th century, there were no dental specialists in orthodontics. All "orthodontia," as it was then called, was done by general dentists. Their appliances were crude, consisting of heavy arch bars to which individual teeth were ligated to produce mostly expansive movements, vulcanite plates, jackscrews, or "cribs" to which were attached "finger" springs. Nevertheless, notable advances during the late 1800s were made by such pioneers as Norman W. Kingsley (1825–1896), John N. Farrar (1839–1913), and Eugene S. Talbot (1847–1925). The "Jackson System," originated by Victor H. Jackson (1850–1929), used such a crib.[1] Bands as we know them today were usually attached only to molars for anchorage purposes.

The idea of "systems" was characteristic of this period of orthodontic history. Each practitioner devised his own method based on purely mechanical considerations and to this system he adhered vehemently. Professional rivalry and dogmatism were the order of the day.

As the century came to a close, there was still no standard orthodontic appliance; no one limited his practice; and there was no school, no journal, nor any society devoted to the specialty. In the dental schools orthodontics was usually lumped in with crown and bridge. For that reason, it received little attention by the deans and faculties of that day.

So it was a time for revolt against the established order. The Filipinos were rebelling against the American occupation. The British were fighting the Boers in South Africa. And the Boxers were besieging a multinational delegation in Peking. Without the bloodshed, but with no less fervor, a group of dedicated dentists brought before the profession the concept that first, the specialty of orthodontics was an area requiring special skills and knowledge and, second, to the mechanical knowledge must be added such basic sciences as anatomy, pathology, and physiology, so that orthodontics could take its place among the learned professions.[2]

CONTRIBUTIONS OF EDWARD H. ANGLE

No one did more to foster orthodontics, to organize, standardize, systematize, and bring about its separation from general practice than did Edward H. Angle (1855–1930). From his experience in teaching at Midwestern dental colleges between 1885 and 1899, he became convinced that, although dentistry and orthodontics both dealt with the human dentition, they were fundamentally different disciplines.[3] Unable to convince authorities of the need for separate curricula, Angle late in 1899 began teaching out of his office in St Louis. It was a humble beginning, with but four students and a course of instruction of only 3 weeks, but by 1927 Angle had trained close to 200 disciples in St Louis, New York City, New London, Connecticut, and Pasadena, California. These graduates were to become the orthodontic department heads (some even became dental school deans) throughout the country, and among the leading researchers and practitioners of the 1900s (the last graduate died in 1993).

This came about not only because of their solid foundation in anatomy, histology, rhinology, embryology, and art during (ultimately) a 1-year course, but because of the fervor of Angle's teaching and the ideals to which he held them. After 1906, he no longer accepted anyone who did not agree to specialize.

Not long after his first classes were under way, Angle organized the American Society (now Association) of Orthodontists. In 1907 he established the first dental specialty journal, *The American Orthodontist*. (Its life was short. The present journal, begun in 1915, is the *American Journal of Orthodontics and Dentofacial Orthopedics*.)

As Angle's graduates took their places in the profession, colleges of dentistry began to appoint them for the teaching of undergraduates, but the courses were still inadequate to prepare them for practicing the demanding specialty. Since the Angle School could not supply the demand for trained orthodontists, other private schools came into being. The first opened in 1907 in St Louis under the name of International School of Orthodontia (1907–1941). It later moved to Kansas City. The second, Dewey School of Orthodontia (1911–ca. 1950), was founded, ironically, by one of Angle's most promising graduates, Martin Dewey. Initially located in Kansas City, the Dewey School ultimately moved to New York.[4]

In addition to his teaching and organizational talents, Angle was a mechanical genius. Beginning with the crude expansion arch prevalent at the time, he developed a series of appliances, each of which offered successively more control and refinement. The heavy arch bar gave way to a precisely formed wire of .022 × .028 inches. The method of fastening to the teeth evolved from simple ligatures to precision slots in brackets welded to precious metal bands cemented to the teeth. With three-dimensional control, clinicians were finally able to achieve bodily tooth movement. The final appliance, perfected 5 years before Angle's death, was given the name edgewise, because the wire's larger dimension was inserted horizontally into the brackets. Today's modified edgewise is the preferred American appliance and is used throughout the world.

Angle's principal legacy was his classification of malocclusion, based on the positions of the first permanent molars. Other classifications have been proffered, but none have been as widely accepted. His most controversial legacy was his stand against tooth extraction. Although initially sanctioning this practice in the case of severely crowded teeth, after witnessing the damage done in the hands of unskilled practitioners, Angle became a passionate opponent of it. So forceful was his stand and so overpowering his personality that few of his disciples dared risk his wrath by opposing him.

One who did frequently disagree with him, though not a disciple, was Calvin S. Case (1847–1923). He attained considerable fame in the designing of appliances for the correction of cleft palate and other oral deformities[5] and was one of the first to recognize the importance of facial esthetics in connection with extraction. Even though Case removed teeth in only 6% of his cases, he was roundly condemned. Only years later was Case accorded his place as one of the greats of orthodontics.

OTHER DEVELOPMENTS TO 1930

The years leading up to the Great Depression were characterized by a steady proliferation of practitioners, the beginnings of graduate training, strong emphasis on mechanics, and an increased interest in biology. Three organizations were formed by Angle's alumni. The first was the short-lived (1906–1913) Alumni Society of the Angle School of Orthodontia. This was followed in 1909 by the Eastern Association of Graduates of the Angle School of Orthodontia, consisting of the New York and New London graduates. It endured for 30 years. In 1922, graduates of Angle's Pasadena school organized the Edward H. Angle Society of Orthodontia, which was a manifestation of the deep influence the school's short term had on them. In the words of Allan G. Brodie, one of its last graduates, "It was a shrine of idealism and like a shrine it drew back those it had sent forth year after year. They came from all parts to have their spirits revived and their ideals burnished bright."[6]

Added to the nearly 200 men and women trained by Angle were graduates of the International and Dewey schools. While not having the reputation of the Angle School (later, College), these schools turned out many orthodontists who achieved distinction. Other specialists were trained by preceptors or by short courses. Although getting a practice started was very slow, eventually most orthodontists enjoyed a high standard of living.

It was not until the early 1920s that dental colleges started adding graduate departments of orthodontics. Up until then, undergraduate courses in that branch of dentistry were scanty and perfunctory. Hands-on training was limited or absent. Many schools closed their clinics because of the lack of interest or failure to produce results.[7] By 1928, four graduate programs had gained a listing in the *Orthodontic Directory of the World*, Forsyth Infirmary, Harvard-Forsyth School, Northwestern University, and the University of Michigan.[8]

By 1925 there were six regional societies, the first having been the Pacific Coast Society of Orthodontists (PCSO), founded in 1913. In 1937, the American Society of Orthodontists became the American Association of Orthodontists (AAO) and incorporated the (then) seven regional (constituent) societies. The eighth and final constituent, the Middle Atlantic Society of Orthodontists, was added in 1952.

During this period, numerous improvements were made in the mechanics of treatment. Charles A. Hawley (1861–1919) introduced the retainer (1908) that bears his name.[9] John V. Mershon (1867–1953) developed the removable lingual arch based on the principle that teeth must be free and unrestricted to adapt to normal growth.[10] In 1928, George Crozat introduced a removable appliance patterned after the Jackson crib. New brackets were designed by James McCoy (1922) and Spencer Atkinson (1929), the latter based on a melding of two of Angle's appliances. Stainless steel was first tried in the late twenties,[11] but it would be 1935 before it achieved clinical application.

Unfortunately, the success of the emerging specialty was not lost on crass commercialism. Casto stated:

> The supply houses and laboratories started an extensive advertising campaign. Standard sets of appliances to meet the requirements of every case were offered to the profession. Laboratories advertised that appliances suitable for use in the treatment of any case would be designed and constructed, either of the fixed or removable type, upon models sent to them by the dentists, at a comparatively small cost. The financial reward appeared attractive, the field fertile, and according to the advertisements the operations were easy and . . . the unscrupulous offered large commissions for the reference patients . . . fundamental principles were disregarded and the science of orthodontia was being prostituted.[12]

Yet there were many whose efforts advanced the science. In the early 1900s, Frederick B. Noyes (1872–1961), an Angle graduate, did important research in dental histology.[13] He later became dental dean at the University of Illinois and one of the most influential leaders in dental education. Benno Lischer (1876–1959), a founder of the International School and later dean and professor of dental orthopedics at Washington University in St Louis, wrote *Principles and Methods of Orthodontia* (1910), in which he advocated early treatment. In 1911, Albin Oppenheim (1875–1945), an Austrian, published his landmark study of tissue changes in orthodontic movement.[14] Alfred Rogers introduced the concept of myofunctional therapy to correct such habits as tongue thrusting, at a time (1918) when other causative factors (such as diet, nutrition, and genetics) were being recognized.

Albert H. Ketcham (1870–1935), devoted researcher and leader of orthodontics in the West, was one of the first to introduce roentgenography and photography into orthodontic diagnosis. He was also instrumental in founding the American Board of Orthodontics (1929), making orthodontics dentistry's first specialty. Another outstanding scientific figure of this period was Milo Hellman (1873–1947). A self-taught anthropologist, Hellman linked the phenomenon of occlusion with the evolution of the dentition as a whole and paved the way for cephalometrics (measurement of living skulls radiographically) by the introduction of craniometry (measurement of dry skulls).[13]

CHAPTER II

From the Depression to the Golden Age (1930-50)

THE 1930s

The year 1930 was a pivotal one for orthodontics. It was, of course, the first year of the Great Depression, which affected the livelihoods of orthodontists as well as others. B. Holly Broadbent was completing his research on the cephalometer, an instrument that accurately positions the head relative to the film and X-ray source.[1] Using this film, or "head plate," the orthodontist was now able to assess the relationship of the teeth to the jaws and the jaws to the face. By the 1950s, cephalometric roentgenography had become a standard diagnostic tool, along with plaster models and photographs.

Though it was the year of Angle's death, it had been 3 years since his college had closed and his followers were concerned about the void it had caused in orthodontic education. Thus, the openings of two important university programs in 1930 were timely. One, organized by George W. Hahn at the University of California, San Francisco, was essentially an undergraduate program that emphasized specialty training during the student's last three years while limiting his or her exposure to other aspects of dentistry. It was called Curriculum II.

The other, at the University of Illinois, was fundamentally a graduate program as were those at Northwestern and Michigan, but, because it had been patterned closely upon Angle's precepts, it soon became the standard for graduate orthodontic education. Under the 36-year direction of Allan Brodie, the University of Illinois became a pioneer in cephalometric research and the fountainhead of future departmental chairpersons throughout the country.

As the depression deepened, orthodontic leaders were concerned about more than economic conditions. Without ignoring advances made by Broadbent and others, Brodie lamented that "orthodontia today is at its lowest ebb. It is held so cheaply by the dental profession that the commercial laboratory is considered fully competent to treat malocclusions," as evidenced by the fact that, in the Middle West, over 80% of general practitioners (GPs) included orthodontics in their services. He reported that three essayists at a recent dental congress independently stated that orthodontics was "retrogressing."[2] The eminent historian Bernhard W. Weinberger also felt that standards of orthodontic practice had degenerated since 1915, citing low educational standards and the

7

increasing frequency of extractions as the chief reasons for the decline. "We are again just where we were 30 or more years ago. These men today merely 'straighten teeth.'"[3]

Leonard Sidlow, who had practiced in Michigan since 1929, recalled, in a February 1986 telephone conversation, "Orthodontics as it was practiced prior to Tweed was in very bad shape. . . . We were finishing cases that were failures. Many of us were at the point where we thought we might give up orthodontics!"

At least technical progress was being made. The introduction of stainless steel in the early 1930s permitted the use of smaller-gauge arch wires, resulting in more comfort for the patient as well as lower cost for components. The use of "stainless" (actually, chrome alloy) allowed orthodontists to weld a variety of attachments to their bands, so the first orthodontic supply companies were organized to meet the growing need. Toward the end of the decade, acrylics were developed for retainers, replacing porous vulcanite, while alginate for impressions was a welcome substitute for the old method of breaking plaster of Paris from the teeth.[4]

Although orthodontic demand was low during the Depression, enough people of means sought treatment for their children to support the existing practitioners, even if it required some traveling to the nearest office.[5] Establishing a branch office and making follow-up phone calls (both common today) were frowned upon and, in fact, the PCSO resolved that "those who indulge in such practices shall be asked to sever their relationship with this organization."[6]

At that time there were very strict dental practice laws, so that formal marketing efforts were virtually unknown. Any such actions were considered unprofessional as well as unethical, and immediate reprimand was certain. Marketing was unstructured and usually consisted of nothing more than joining the Rotary or taking local dentists to lunch. However, after a long period of building one's reputation, the established orthodontist reigned supreme in his area and presented a formidable obstacle to any newcomer attempting to start a practice.[5]

Early Advertisers

Unfortunately, such strictures did not prevent nonmembers of organized dentistry from hawking their wares. The first orthodontic advertisement to appear in the Los Angeles Classified Section was placed in 1935 by general dentist Leo James Grold (USC '25).[7] (Advertising, according to ethical dentists, was proffering one's name before the public in any but the most conservative manner. This would include, but not be limited to, print and electronic media, billboards, office signs, stationery, and business cards. In the case of yellow page advertising, it would include printing any announcement more conspicuous than the customary unbolded listing.)

Advertisers were not new to Los Angeles. When Painless Parker, the "father of advertising dentists," moved to L.A. in 1906, he counted eight advertisers in the downtown area.[8] In the 1930s and '40s, the biggest advertisers were credit dentists such as Dr Campbell and Dr Beauchamp, who offered "dental plates" on a pay-later basis.[9]

In fact, dental advertising is as old as dentistry itself. Prior to the early 1800s, it was considered good professional form and was customary among all health practitioners.[10] Early attempts to curb advertising in the dental profession did not arise until the first American dental society, the Society of Dental Surgeons of the City and State of New York, was formed in 1834. Even so, the ban could apply only to the society's members—as is true today. Although most state dental practice laws forbad advertising by state-registered dentists, they were rarely enforced.[11] The PCSO expressed its concern in 1938 when it proclaimed: "Advertising dentists are propagandizing the public on orthodontic treatment. Unqualified persons are soliciting orthodontic practice under the guise of 'school clinics.' Newspapers, phone books, pamphlets, and even neon signs blazon the words that teeth are 'straightened.'"[12]

Harbinger of the Future

But it was not necessary to advertise in order to build a large, efficient practice. The most advanced orthodontic office of the day (started in the '20s) was that of James and John McCoy of Los Angeles. It occupied the entire floor of their own building on Wilshire Boulevard and featured four operatories (two for each doctor), a reception lobby, a business office/library for each doctor, a laboratory, an X-ray/photography room, a kitchenette, dressing rooms, even a patio. As soon as one patient was finished, the doctor would move to his other room, where another patient was waiting—a forerunner of today's routine. However, this facility was a marked exception. The typical office was not geared to production. It consisted simply of one or two chairs and a girl Friday, who acted as receptionist, chair side assistant, and lab technician. All patient procedures were done by the doctor, usually standing, with the assistant sometimes mixing cement, handing instruments, or taking X-rays.[13]

Mail-Order Orthodontics

The practice of mail-order orthodontics also continued to vex orthodontic leaders. Leuman M. Waugh, former president of the AAO, said,

"The most untenable and harmful of these [practices] is the orthodontic appliance designed and made in the dental laboratory. . . . It has no inherent intelligence and can act only as mechanically directed." But he allowed that the laboratories were less to be blamed than those dentists who patronized them.[14] In writing to the advertising manager of a popular dental journal, Paul G. Spencer, representing the Southwestern Society of Orthodontists, stated, "Certainly no conscientious publisher of medical literature would advise the embryo surgeon to seek instruction about how to perform an operation from the mechanic who makes surgical instruments."[15] The PCSO called it "a form of dental quackery."[16] Almost 30 years were to elapse before the AAO was able to exercise some control over this practice when, in 1963, it gained representation on the Joint Commission Accreditation of Dental Laboratories of the American Dental Association.[17]

Despite the depressed economic conditions of the '30s and the encroachment of nonorthodontists onto his turf, the typical specialist enjoyed the good life: He could practice without government interference (other than maintaining his state license and paying taxes); he could set his own fees; his office was a cottage and not a clinic; and he answered to no one except himself, his patients, and his ethics committee.

WORLD WAR II AND POSTWAR YEARS

On January 25, 1945, eight months before the war's end, Grand Rapids, Michigan, became the first city in the world to fluoridate its water supply. Thus began the era of fluoridation, which was to have a profound effect on dental practice and ultimately on orthodontics.[18]

The war did not impede the efforts being made in clinical and theoretical research. The work of Charles H. Tweed (1895–1970) had probably the greatest impact on clinical orthodontic practice of the 1940s and many years beyond. The result was that facial esthetics gained new importance in diagnosis, and extraction treatment was taken out of the "closet"; Tweed's office in Tucson, Arizona, became a mecca for those seeking to learn his technique.

In theoretical research at the University of Illinois, Brodie completed in 1941 an 8-year study of the growth patterns of the human head.[19] William B. Downs (1899–1966), a protégé of Brodie's, published his cephalometric analysis of the facial skeleton in 1948, effectively putting an end to the "era of model diagnosis."[20] A Danish orthodontist, Arne Björk, made a significant contribution to basic research in facial growth with the publication of his book, *The Face in Profile* (1947).[21]

Early Clinics

The war years also saw the appearance of a new phenomenon: the clinic. The first commercial orthodontic clinic known to this author was that of Merle C. Brooks (USC '32), near the University of Southern California in 1945.[22] Brooks was a general dentist, but nothing prevented him, according to California law, from practicing orthodontics. Nor did it keep him from hiring other dentists to do so.

There has been a great deal of ambiguity associated with the word *clinic*. Webster defines it as "(1) a facility (as of a hospital) for diagnosis and treatment of outpatients, or (2) a group practice which several physicians work cooperatively."[23] Clinics can be institutional or private, nonprofit or for profit, medical or dental. However, you will not find a listing of "Dental Clinics" in the Los Angeles yellow pages. This may be an indication of the pejorative connotation dental professionals have hung on the term.

An example of a nonpejorative use of clinic is the group of facilities (then 11) founded in 1946 by the Los Angeles Dental Society and local PTA in response to closure of the public school-financed clinics. Reflecting the state board's requirement that they be operated as a private practice, the clinics have been known since 1953 by the name Robert L. Taylor (originally Harold W. Barnes), DDS, Dental Clinics (now Clinic). A full range of pediatric dental services is offered Los Angeles school children, but no orthodontics.[24]

According to a New Jersey bill signed in June 1951, a dental clinic is "any clinic, infirmary, hospital, institution or other place of any kind whatsoever, in which the science of dentistry in any of its branches is practiced, demonstrated or taught . . . but shall not include the private office of a regularly licensed dentist of this state."[25] For the purpose of this history, an orthodontic clinic is one designed to offer treatment at low cost and to maximize the flow of patients, using production methods, including one or more of the following: (1) multiple chairs (up to 20 or 25), (2) doctors (often multiple) employed on either a salary or per diem basis, and (3) chairside assistants performing the maximum number of procedures permitted by law (after 1974).

Some private clinics were started for humanitarian reasons: to bring orthodontic treatment within reach of families who could not otherwise afford it. Others were run strictly for profit. Most had elements of both. It is not known what the motivation was behind some of the earlier Los Angeles clinics, but there is no question that their owners did well. According to Henry Levin, a pedodontist who worked about a year for Brooks, the clinic grossed almost $500,000 in 1958. This estimate is based on a patient load of 150 per day, each paying $12.50 a month (after a down payment of $45), and being seen every 2 weeks.

The dentists were paid $50 per day, considered generous for those days, but their training was limited. Henry Levin, in a telephone conversation with the author in June 1995, recalled, "My job was to pinch bands, spot weld them, and solder them." When asked how he learned to do this, he replied, "You watched the guy next to you." Henry Duim (USC '38), a supervisor, was "a marvelous practitioner," according to Robert J. Flynn, another Brooks "alumnus," in a phone conversation with the author in June 1995. "I used to follow him around like a puppy dog and take every course I could think of." But dentists who worked for Brooks were barred from the dental society.

As for results, Flynn noted that they were both good and bad. Levin was more critical. "People mainly wanted their six front teeth straight. That was the only purpose I could remember. There were very few who came out of there with a Class I [normal occlusion]."

The war itself had two main effects on the orthodontic specialty. First, mobilization created a temporary shortage of specialists. In 1944, almost 12% of the 746 AAO members were in the service.[26] This group not only had to close their offices (unless special arrangements could be made with associates), but they were also unable to ply their trade in the dental dispensaries because straight teeth were not deemed essential in combat. The remaining 88% were swamped with patients.

Second, returning dentists, with their careers already interrupted and the G.I. Bill in hand to cover costs, saw their discharge as an opportunity to enroll in graduate programs before returning to practice. Orthodontic programs soon had long waiting lists. At the same time, demand for orthodontic services increased with the postwar prosperity and the enlightenment of parents about treatment. Thus, many new graduate departments were organized throughout the country during the 1950s and '60s and fledgling orthodontists were turned out in larger and larger numbers. These university graduates had no problem finding new, busy, and profitable locations.[27]

During these decades, research thrived, textbooks were published, principles of biomechanics became better understood, new materials greatly improved what appliances could do, and new functional appliances (one- or two-piece appliances, often removable, designed to change the jaw relationship and/or muscle pressures) were introduced. Through the joint efforts of orthodontists and maxillofacial surgeons, along with new and daring techniques (perfected in the '70s), correction of hitherto "hopeless" cases became possible through jaw surgery.[28]

CHAPTER III

The Golden Age (1950–70)

From around 1950 to 1970, the specialty of orthodontics was bathed in prosperity. The postwar baby boom that had started in 1946 was in full swing. Between 1954 and 1957 (the peak year), more than 4 million babies were born each year in the United States.[1] And since there still were relatively few practitioners, most of them had a waiting list of 2 years. In California, backlogs of 12 months were not uncommon. In a telephone interview February 1996, C.W. "Clu" Carey of Palo Alto stated that he had a waiting list of two years. Lawrence L. Furstman, a Beverly Hills orthodontist, recalled in a phone conversation with the author in December 1987 that, "In 1960 . . . these kids could get out of school and be making big money within 6 months because there was such a crying need in areas like Orange County . . ." In 1962, AAO president Dallas R. McCauley called the supply of graduate orthodontic departments in dental schools "inadequate."[2]

The specialty's leaders thought the bonanza would never end. As late as 1965, they even expected an increase in the demand for orthodontic care. Melvin Dollar, lay executive director of the New York State Dental Service Corporation, predicted that "the rapidly increasing number of children in the population, coupled with continuing prosperity, is likely to bring a more immediate surge of demand for orthodontic care . . . immediate attention should be given to expanding the number of orthodontists and introducing new methods to increase the orthodontists' capacity to handle more cases."[3]

As a consequence of these expectations, from 1967 to 1974 the number of orthodontic students being trained at the university level rose from 469 to 685. In addition, the AAO inaugurated a preceptorship program in 1958 whereby a dentist could train in the office of an approved preceptor for a period of 3 years, during which he or she would receive didactic, as well as on-the-job, training. This self-limiting program was to be arbitrarily terminated by January 1, 1967. Individuals accepted before the cutoff date would have until 1970 to complete their training. In the 11 years of its existence, the preceptorship program produced 266 orthodontists.[4,5]

The specialty, responding to a need, had met that need. But had they met it too well?

PREPAID DENTISTRY

One of the reasons the profession was lulled into a false sense of security was the constant increase of private prepaid and government-funded dental programs that were expected to bring about a "spectacular rise" in the demand for orthodontic treatment."[6] As early as 1936, *American Journal of Orthodontics (AJO)* editor Harvey C. Pollack Jr had warned, "Medical and dental service for larger groups of people is not on the way; it is now here... . Orthodontists . . . must realize that this very thing is now happening in a more or less slow motion tempo but will gain momentum from year to year."[7] By 1966, more than 3 million persons were covered by 525 dental prepayment programs, and that figure was expected to reach 15 million by 1970.[8] Of 22 companies that insured for dental care, 16 included orthodontic treatment; however, only one of these companies specified the educational qualifications of the provider-dentist.[9]

Although the majority of AAO members were initially in favor of exploring prepaid orthodontic programs, F. Gene Dixon, vice-president and managing director of the California Dental Association Service, voiced the concern of many dentists with regard to prepayment plans when he warned that one of the greatest dangers is control from outside the profession.[10] Accordingly, the AAO adopted in 1967 a policy statement that stressed, among other things, that (1) whenever possible the third party in dental care programs be a dental service corporation; (2) primary importance be placed on the quality of treatment; (3) treatment be rendered only by qualified orthodontists; and (4) patients have a free choice of doctor.[11] The AAO also urged the formation of an official state orthodontic society in every state, to be available as consultants to state dental service corporations concerning prepayment problems.[12] The development of insurance plans through dental service corporations was regarded as the profession's best weapon against third-party control because, according to the general secretary of the American Dental Association (ADA), not only would the profession itself benefit from operating its own plans, but there was a public need for such plans and a tendency for government to move into areas of unmet need.[13]

However, it was one thing for an organization to state its policy, quite another for commercial interests to follow it. PCSO president Donald E. Priewe complained that solicitors of prepaid plans engaged in mass mailings and "do not even have the courtesy of presenting the proposal to . . . the California State Society of Orthodontists for consideration."[14]

PANELS

Labor unions also began adding dental, and eventually, orthodontic benefits to their health plans as members got caught up in the trend toward demanding health care benefits. This demand led to (1) the establishment of clinics to provide care under union ownership or (2) the union's contracting with private dental offices—usually a group practice—for such care. These facilities, or panels, took one or both of the following forms: In the closed panel, benefits were paid only if treatment was provided by a dentist who had agreed to the terms of the plan, one of which was a reduced fee. The number of dentists in a given panel area was to be limited. In an open panel, beneficiaries could choose any licensed dentist to provide their care, although the dentist was under no contractual obligation to treat any patient, with payments made either to the dentist or directly to the patient.[15] In July 1996, dental consultant Jay W. Friedman reported in a telephone interview that most open panel plans required a copayment of 20% to 50%, except for records (X-rays, photographs, and models). The panel concept would be adopted in the 1970s by insurance companies.

The first union-sponsored group practice in the Los Angeles area—and the first capitated dental plan for children—was the Wilmington (later Harbor City), California, practice of Max H. Schoen. It was organized for the purpose of providing services for members of the International Longshoremen's and Warehousemen's Union (ILWU).[16] (Outsiders and those who were employed by Schoen commonly referred to the facility as "the clinic," but the term was never used by Schoen and his partners.) Opening in 1954, the group began accepting orthodontic patients about 2 years later. Schoen's group had characteristics of both the closed and open panel, providing services on both a fee-for-service and capitation basis.[17] The fee-for-service component, now Delta Dental, was called the California Dental Service Group. A similar group practice was located in San Francisco. ILWU's efforts stimulated the development of service corporations (by the dental societies) to administer these programs.[18] Critics of prepaid care were probably surprised to learn that examiners gave the clinic a clean bill of health, finding that the services were "consistently above average."[19]

It wasn't long before the group had broadened its base to include patients from all walks of life. Part-time orthodontists were paid $75 per day; full-time, $1,000 a month. Since each clinician was assigned only one chair and one assistant, there was no pressure to increase production. Recent graduates such as Ruth D. Carter, who spent about 2 years with the group in the late 1950s, looked on the clinic as a place where they could obtain an immediate income—as well as gain valuable experience— while seeking to start a practice of their own. To the established practitioner, however, it was a threat. "Everyone felt that they were being threatened, because that was a segment of the population that would not be coming to them," said Carter in a telephone interview with the author in July 1995.

However, it is debatable whether these patients constituted a potential market for mainstream orthodontists. Raymond W. Weinshenker, a contemporary of Carter's, believed not. He said, during a telephone interview in July 1995, "It was a trade-off. They were somewhat of a threat. But patients who were going to the Longshoreman's, for example, wouldn't have been able to get any treatment." He did, however, concur that organized dentistry's attitude toward any kind of prepaid care was "horrible." Even more "horrible" was its attitude toward advertisers.

The editor of a constituent society dental bulletin wrote that "the majority of dentists in Southern California considered the new breed of advertising dentist who sets up a closed panel clinic and makes a contract with a group for dental care . . . at a discount price to be highly unethical." Society members were surprised that better-educated groups such as the San Diego County Employee's Association and other municipal groups were not better informed about how limited their dental care could be under a closed panel contract.[20] In November 1967 the ADA, at its annual meeting, voiced its opposition to closed panels because of the "essential limitation which this method of practice imposes on the patient."[21]

But Dr Matthew L. Prescott, director of a cooperative dental clinic in Milwaukee, Wisconsin, that opened in August 1965 under the terms of a union contract, argued that closed panels provide quality dental care for people who most need it and can least afford it. To back up his claim, he cited the fact that, in its first 2 years of operation, the clinic had treated several thousand adults who had not visited a dentist in at least 5 years and had established a dental care program for thousands of youngsters who had never visited a dentist in their lives. He further claimed that the real gripe of panel opponents was the fear of losing patients.[22]

In rebuttal, Martin B. Robbins of Phoenix, Arizona, maintained that the basic idea of a closed panel clinic is socialistic. He did not dispute the fact that people using clinics would not otherwise get adequate care, but argued that patients seek care not because of the clinic, but because of the insurance. Studies have shown that, where subscribers are allowed to buy dental insurance or get it paid for by their employer or unions, they tend to use the facilities of private practitioners just as well. He also wondered what would happen when inflation drives up costs. Would clinic directors raise salaries, or will they sacrifice quality by cutting corners and driving operators "to work faster and sloppier"?[23]

THE GRAVY TRAIN

Around 1960 there was a rekindling of GP interest in orthodontics. This was brought about not only by their awareness of the specialists' prosperity, but by a drop in their own busyness as a result of the increasing prevalence of fluoridation, a downturn in the economy (starting in the late fifties), and a coincidental downtrend in the birthrate (having peaked in 1957). In addition, the popularity of removable appliances, traditionally used by Europeans, was spreading to the United States and generalists saw removables as involving less time and risk than fixed ones.[24]

Goading them on, as in the 1930s, were the mail-order orthodontic laboratories, who invited GPs to "cash in on the orthodontic boom," as one flyer proclaimed. "Just send us your models and . . . we will even send instructions on how to adjust the appliances."[25]

Of course, not all general dentists were after a quick buck. To be sure, a large segment of the out-group was genuinely interested in providing a professional service for the many malocclusion cases they saw on a daily basis. Legally, they could do it, but they wanted more knowledge. If they wanted to do more endodontics (root canals), for instance, they could take refresher courses. The same held true for pedodontics, oral surgery, and other specialties. Those specialties had graduate programs and board certification just as did orthodontics, but nobody even said boo if GPs undertook such procedures in their offices. Why then, nonspecialists asked, were orthodontists the only group up in arms over dentists' putting braces on their own patients?

If periodontists, endodontists, and prosthodontists (crown and bridge specialists) have responded differently to GPs, it may be that these groups have found their disciplines to be more amenable to generalist and specialist divisions of treatment that do not result in two different levels of care.[26]

Generalists complained that "courses are practically unavailable to all but 'recognized' specialists. Educational facilities are closely guarded and controlled. Only in our specialty has the withholding of education from those who seek it become an acceptable procedure, while courses in all other branches of dentistry are made available to all who wish to participate."[27] Typical of the gibes was the one hurled at one of the specialty's leading teachers and researchers, during an interdisciplinary staff meeting: "Hey, Rick, what are you orthodontists going to hold over us when we learn everything about cephalometrics?"[28]

Responsible members of the in-group sympathized with their nonspecialist brethren but tried to make it clear that orthodontics was a completely different ball game. It was more than just taking a few extra months of training. It was virtually a profession unto itself, as Angle had so often proclaimed. The best way to deal with the situation, according to AAO president Dallas R. McCauley, was to educate the general dentists in their undergraduate curriculum. "The more every dentist knows of the biologic and physiologic aspects of the growing and developing orodental complex, the more he will respect the difficulties of orthodontic therapy."[29] And who is more hesitant to undertake unsupervised treatment than a graduate student 6 months or so into training? They have learned enough to recognize their ignorance.

For the moment, however, nonspecialists were more impressed with demographics than with biology. As late as 1974, the ADA estimated that "the number of persons needing orthodontic care will almost double (from 4.0 million in 1970 to 7.6 million in 1990) . . . It is apparent that the manpower will not be sufficient." Therefore, the Academy of General Dentistry urged that the profession train more general dentists and pedodontists to provide essential orthodontic services.[30] Unfortunately, the profession failed to realize that it is not need that creates patients—it is demand.

In 1958, the *Journal of Dentistry for Children* published an article entitled "How Much Orthodontics Shall the Pedodontist Do?,"[31] reflecting the confusion that existed—and still exists—between the two specialties. Since then, numerous conferences and workshops among the specialties and the ADA have been held to define boundaries, but little progress has been made. During the 1976 workshop, for example, the position of the AAO was that "when orthodontic care is provided by a specialist, that specialist should be an orthodontist, and that pedodontics be limited to prevention of malocclusion including space maintenance and minor space recovery and preventive orthodontic measures that do not involve existing orthodontic problems."[32]

But due to fluoridation's effect on cavities, the "birth dearth," an increase in the number of pedodontists, and increasing intrusions into their bailiwick by general practitioners, "the orthodontic specialty was experiencing ever-increasing incursions . . . from the pedodontist who is redefining his practice and establishing broader educational guidelines.[11]

LAWSUITS

Orthodontics' golden age was further tarnished in the early '60s by the efforts of two dentists who, after failing to gain admission to the PCSO, separately sued the society and its parent body, the AAO.[34] The first suit was brought in 1961 by Leon J. Pinsker of Lakewood, California. Pinsker was qualified by virtue of his education, but he was refused membership on the grounds that he practiced with an unqualified partner (Max Schleimer). He sued the PCSO, the AAO, and their officers in 1961, seeking to compel his admission. The litigation was protracted for a period of 10 years, including three reviews by the state supreme court.[35] The final verdict was that Pinsker must be admitted if he qualified under the current rules, but by the time he was admitted to the society in 1976, he had founded his own association, according to Warren A. Kitchen, in a telephone interview by the author in November 1994.

The second action was brought by Bertram Kronen, a Santa Rosa, California, dentist who contended that the societies had conspired to deny him active membership and had refused to consider his application "willfully or without right." The trial court found that the dentist was not properly qualified, had not complied with the by-laws, and did not have proper endorsers for his application (recommendations were withheld because of his lack of competency, his poor relations with patients and colleagues, and his refusal to let the endorsers visit his office). The court's findings were upheld by the First District Court of Appeal (California), which found that "the activities of (the defendants) . . . emanated not from conspiracy, as claimed by the plaintiff, but from a sincere sense of responsibility to their profession, the public and even to the plaintiff himself."[36]

SPLINTER GROUPS

Barred from admission to the orthodontic societies and unable to attend a university graduate program without giving up their livelihood for 2 or more years, orthodontic wannabes set up their own professional associations for the purpose of not only breaking down barriers to graduate orthodontic training, but for recognition as specialists and the publication of their own journals. One of the first such associations was the New York Society for the Study of Orthodontics, founded in 1945 by 15 alumni of the Neustadt Institute of Orthodontics. They hoped to gain knowledge by, among other things, inviting eminent orthodontists to lecture.

But it wasn't long before the group ran afoul of mainstream orthodontists, with the discovery that one of the by-laws of the New York Society of Orthodontists (NYSO), a component of the AAO and the group from which lecturers would be drawn, "disapproves of the members . . . participating in any capacity before an orthodontic society that is not recognized by the American Association of Orthodontists." Only after a strenuous letter-writing campaign and political maneuvering within the local dental society, did the out-group compel the NYSO to rescind its proscriptive rule.[37]

The first splinter group to achieve widespread notice was the International Academy (now Association) of Orthodontics (IAO), founded in 1961 in California, by Max Schleimer and Leon Pinsker, the latter becoming its first president.[38] Within a year of its founding, the association's journal, the *International Journal of Orthodontics (IJO)* (not to be confused with the old *International Journal of Orthodontia, etc.*), started featuring Pinsker's scathing editorials. Calling orthodontics the "sacred cow of dentistry"[39] and a "key club,"[40] and referring to the AAO's restrictive policies as "the stainless steel curtain," Pinsker called for complete educational freedom and increased facilities for the training of graduate orthodontists. He further proposed that the ADA Council of Dental Education "meet in an emergency session to consider the extreme shortage of orthodontists in this country."[41]

Flak was also received from other quarters. The First District Dental Society of the State of New York accused orthodontists of "trying to stifle the teaching of the specialty." The ADA, through its Council on Dental Education, agreed that "admission to continuing education courses in special areas of practice should be based upon specific educational prerequisites, rather than on membership in a particular specialty society."[42]

Responding to the pressure, AAO President Earl E. Shepard in 1964 admitted, "We have certainly been accused of erecting . . . a means of preventing worthwhile knowledge from emanating to the general practitioner . . . certain citadels of learning have used membership in our organization as a means of accepting or rejecting applicants . . ." Section 23 of the association's code of ethics was rescinded.[43]

Apparently this did not satisfy the needs of IAO members. In 1970, Robert W. Donovan, one of IAO's organizers and editor-in-chief of the *IJO*, opened the United States Dental Institute (USDI) in Chicago to offer GPs and pedodontists more comprehensive training in orthodontics than was then available by way of short courses. AAO members could hardly be blamed for feeling a sense of betrayal when they learned that Donovan was not only a university-trained orthodontist who had been on the Northwestern University faculty, but had received the first PhD in orthodontics ever awarded by that institution.[44]

Three or four years after the opening, the ADA, the AAO, the Illinois Dental Society, and the Illinois Society of Orthodontists filed a formal complaint with the state's superintendent of public instruction seeking to have USDI's accreditation as a postsecondary educational institution revoked.[45] The USDI and 10 dentists promptly filed a class action suit (October 1974) against the ADA, the AAO, individual officers, and others, alleging an antitrust violation and a conspiracy to prevent general dentists from becoming orthodontists. They asked for damages of $85.2 million.[46]

Commenting on the suit, C. Gordon Watson, executive director of the ADA, said that "if the United States Dental Institute were ever upheld in this action, the national dental educational standards . . . would be seriously undermined."[47] Four years later, after numerous hearings, USDI agreed to dismiss its suit. Concurrently the Illinois Office of Education ruled that USDI could continue to operate solely as an institute of continuing education.[48]

The decline of the golden age of orthodontics was the decline of more than economic plenty. It also marked the end of what might be called the "conservative" period. The specialty was still under the influence of conscientious leaders who tried to instill a philosophy of high treatment standards and professionalism. During this era, practice management courses were practically unknown because emphasis was focused entirely on technically excellent results. Since the orthodontist performed most of his or her own procedures, the number of patients seen in a day was limited. Most practices did not treat more than 100 to 120 patients at any given time, and fees and expectations were modest.[49]

A few sounded warnings. William S. Parker of the *PCSO Bulletin* editorialized:

> Unless an unforeseen economic bonanza occurs it is not hard to see that all of these forces and facts will come together at a point in the not-too-distant future with untold consequences. . . . Meantime we follow the same formats and have pleasant meetings attended by a faithful few. It is just possible that we should be arranging some very serious workshop-type meetings to consider this juxtaposition of facts which is now being mixed to produce a witch's brew.[50]

No single event or proclamation marked the end of the golden age. Those who reaped from it were probably not even aware of its existence. Like other eras of history, it would take hindsight to recognize it. But as waiting lists disappeared, as competition increased, and as choice locations in the suburbs became filled, it did not take a psychic to see that the halcyon days of orthodontics were reaching an end.

CHAPTER IV

Decline (1970–80s)

Reacting to the growing unrest among its constituents, the American Association of Orthodontists conducted a manpower survey in 1972. For the first time, the official body admitted that all was not well:

> There is no doubt that orthodontic practices have definitely leveled off from previous experiences. While not clearly defined in this survey, a possibility exists that the influx of orthodontists into cities or metropolitan areas may have caused unusual competition among orthodontists themselves and/or with general practitioners.

While admitting that "orthodontic practice growth does not look too bright in the near future," the analysts pointed out that population is not the only determinant of practice "health." Personal income, better geographic distribution of orthodontists, public education, relationship with GPs, and the amount of orthodontics done by GPs were also important criteria. But all these factors were cause for concern. When asked to pinpoint the major reason for their "unbusyness," the respondents answered:

Too many new orthodontists	54%
Economic conditions (recession)	30%
Competition with general practitioners	14%
Other	41%[1]

In 1974 AAO president Hubert J. Bell cautioned that "we seem to have more and greater problems facing our specialty now than at any time in our history. One of the most perplexing problems is the continuous and explosive appearance of various courses, short and long, giving the nonorthodontist training in orthodontics." Unfortunately, the association "is not a regulatory body, and we can only police our own membership."[2]

FORCES OUTSIDE ORTHODONTICS

The Birthrate

The single most detrimental force acting on orthodontics in the sixties and seventies was the declining birthrate. After peaking in 1957, the birthrate underwent a 15-year decline, dropping in 1972 to its lowest level (2.03 children per mother) in American history. The FDA approved the first oral contraceptive ("the pill") in 1960, which had a major impact on the fertility rate. In 1976, the number of births per 1000 women of child-bearing age was 65—only half of what it was in the peak year.[3] Factoring in the anticipated orthodontist population, the *Journal of Clinical Orthodontics* *(JCO)* predicted that the ratio of 12-year-olds to orthodontists would drop from the 1950 figure of about 2000 to 400 by 1982.[4] In Illinois, total school enrollment peaked in 1971 and by 1973 had started a slow decline.[5] In 1975, the Pacific Coast had the least desirable child-per-orthodontist ratio (320) compared with other AAO constituents, while at the same time it was experiencing the next-to-largest rate of increase of orthodontists starting practice.[6]

President D. Robert Swineherd told the Middle Atlantic Society of Orthodontists that "the demand for our individual services has decreased in arithmetical, if not algebraic, proportions." Northeastern Society President Nicholas A. DiSalvo wistfully commented, "Gone are the good old days when all one had to do was to unlock his office door and pick patients off the waiting line." Worst of all the eight regional societies, as reported in the survey, was the PCSO, with only 52.1% reporting that they were even moderately busy, compared with the national average of 63%. "The situation is so severe in California that some recent orthodontic graduates have turned to general practice in order to keep from having to leave the field of dentistry entirely."[6]

Legislation

Advertising. Until the mid-70s, advertising by dentists was prohibited by many state dental practice acts and, according to the ADA, was a breach of professional ethics. But in 1975 the Supreme Court ruled in *Goldfarb vs Virginia State Bar* that there was no "learned professions" exception to antitrust laws and that, therefore, they apply with full vigor to the activities of professional associations. Thus, an association prohibiting advertising by its members was looked upon as restraint of trade. Two years later the court sounded the death knell of the 110-year prohibition. In the case of *Bates and O'Steen vs State Bar of Arizona*, it ruled that it was restraint of trade for the legal profession to restrict advertising by its members. As a result of these rulings, the ADA and the Federal Trade Commission (FTC) entered a consent decree in 1979 to allow dentists to advertise.[7]

In its opinion, the High Court wrote, "Advertising serves to inform the public of the availability, nature, and prices of products and services, and thus performs an indispensable role in the allocation of resources in a free enterprise system."[7] The AAO immediately adopted resolutions to comport with the rulings, saying that "there is no bar to membership of an orthodontist who advertises provided that such advertisement is consistent with government restriction, particularly, and does not contain anything which may be presumed to be false or misleading."[8] Younger practitioners apparently took these new developments in stride. However, older orthodontists who had begun in a different era viewed these efforts with concern and uneasiness, fearing the rise of crass commercialism. Formerly, their colleagues were their best friends; now they were viewed suspiciously as competitors trying to take away their market share.[9]

Putting it more bluntly, a public relations man for a Long Island dental clinic said, "What advertising has done is transformed dentistry into a product, rather than a service. And, as everyone knows, with a product you shop around—and, if you're typical, you buy price."[10] In the Los Angeles yellow pages, ads for orthodontics (anything larger than standard listings) jumped from 2 in 1975 to 16 in 1980. All except one were made by general dentists who hired specialists to handle the orthodontic portion of their practice.[11]

Even the hard-earned master's degree (customarily granted to those graduate students completing a thesis) came under attack. The judicial council of the California Dental Association (CDA) notified AAO components that the MS, MSD, and the PhD "are nonspecific. Certainly they do not inform the public of any particular skill in any particular area of dentistry."[12]

Aid to education, facilities, and incorporation. Starting in the early 1960s, the federal government became more and more involved in health care. Fully aware of the nation's shortage of providers, its initial efforts were directed to increase the opportunities for training of professional health personnel. Calling the nation's medical and dental schools "a national resource," Congress passed the Health Professions Educational Assistance Act of 1963, providing construction, loans, and other aid to schools and students. ADA President Gerald D. Timmons called it "well-conceived and critically needed health legislation."[13]

As time went on, however, legislation was geared less to relieving shortages and more to making health care accessible to lower income groups. In 1976 Congress passed the Public Health Service Act. Title VII of this act, authorizing $136.1 million in capitation grants to schools of dentistry and other health sciences and more than $1.5 million in loans to graduate students, was designed to flood the market with enough health care practitioners to alleviate the shortage in remote areas and to bring down the cost of care.[14] By now it was clear to the professions that all this largesse was beginning to break their backs, and the ADA leadership was singing a different tune. President Carlton H. Williams referred to the involvement as "encroachment of government in our affairs," and "an inordinate interest in health care."[15]

Nor did this largesse come free. Railroads, aircraft companies, the postal service, farmers, the poor—they all received subsidies, but Amtrak, for instance, was not expected to lower its fares because of them. Yet people outside the profession saw the subsidies (their tax money), increased production, and use of expanded duty auxiliaries as justification to lower fees.[16]

Other far-reaching laws allowed professionals to incorporate. After a series of test cases over the years involving physicians' groups claiming the right to be taxed as corporations, the federal government finally decided to let the states determine whether an entity was a corporation. The states responded by adopting legislation permitting professionals to incorporate. In 1968, California became the 37th state to do so.[17] Though these laws were welcomed by dentists wanting to take advantage of the profit-sharing and pension plans, tax write-offs, and other features, their detrimental effect was the encouragement they gave to the formation of multiple clinic operations. Clinics were further encouraged by Title V of PL 89-754 (1966), which provided mortgage insurance for group practice facilities and placed the solo practitioner at an economic disadvantage.[18]

Title XI of the National Housing Act authorized FHA loans to qualified group practices for new construction, expansion, or remodeling. In its booklet on the program, the Department of Urban Development states: "b. Group practice makes possible more efficient use of *scarce manpower* [author's emphasis] . . ."[19]

Extended functions. Even more influential in terms of large-scale operations were laws giving dental auxiliaries "extended functions." In California, Assembly Bill (AB)1455 was signed into law on April 2, 1974.[20] The State Board of Dental Examiners spelled out the regulations: Trained and licensed registered dental assistants (RDAs) would be allowed, under doctor supervision, to perform such procedures as the taking of diagnostic records, fitting of bands and removable appliances, removal and tying in (adjusted) archwires, removal of cement, and giving instructions to the patient in oral hygiene and the care of appliances.[21]

To those orthodontic practitioners who were unable to accommodate all the patients seeking care (a rarity by now), these regulations allowed them to see more patients in a given day. To those less busy, the change meant that they would now have more time to spend on administrative matters, such as case analysis, or they could play more golf. But to union leaders, insurance company executives, and ambitious GPs, it meant lower-cost treatment for large numbers of patients who heretofore could not afford it. They envisioned spacious, modern clinics where hired orthodontists would walk up and down the line, giving instructions to highly skilled auxiliaries doing 90% of the work.

The idea of extended duties in orthodontic practice was not new, having been used by two Maryland orthodontists, Harold E. Eskew and Harry S. Galblum, in the 1950s. Both were members of the Edward H. Angle Society of Orthodontia (a prestigious group having strict membership requirements) and were board certified. Borrowing ideas from Robert W. Donovan of Chicago, they set up separate practices where up to 80 patients could be seen in one day by one doctor (although associate orthodontists were the rule). Speaking to groups throughout the country, Eskew and Galblum might be called the pioneers of production methods in orthodontics (according to telephone interviews with F.H. Wallace and Galblum, respectively, in August 1997.

Continuing education. In an effort to ensure continued competence of practicing dentists, the California Legislature in 1972 passed AB 1442, requiring that, effective May 1, 1974, all dentists renewing their licenses must have completed 50 hours of approved continuing education (CE) courses during the prior 2 years.[22] Since these courses were not free, many dentists looked at the requirement as an imposition on their time and pocketbooks. Orthodontists attending scientific sessions during regular meetings could now receive a certain number of CE credits. Practitioners could also sign up for correspondence courses, or even listen to audiotapes while driving to their offices. Thus a whole new industry grew up marketing courses to doctors.

Burakoff and Demby, in a report on quality assurance, did not support the concept of mandatory continuing education. "Although the use of continuing education is expanding, there is little hard evidence of its efficiency in promoting competence."[23] In California, the number of cases of incompetence and unprofessional conduct appearing before the dental boards did not seem to have diminished in the 23 years of the law's existence. And the malpractice lawyers were busier than ever.

Infection control. Concern for worker safety had existed for more than 2000 years. As early as the fourth century BC Hippocrates recognized and recorded problems associated with exposure to lead in mining. About 400 years later, Pliny the Elder discussed the dangers in handling zinc and sulfur. Laws to enforce worker protection began to appear around the world in the 18th and 19th centuries. By 1948, all the states had workmen's compensation laws.[24] In 1970, Congress passed the Occupational Safety and

Health Act (OSHA), to protect workers from hazards in the workplace. About half the states, including California (Cal/OSHA), have opted to institute their own OSHA programs.

Although dentists have always been subject to OSHA, it was not until 1983, when the Centers for Disease Control (CDC) in Atlanta announced the discovery of AIDS, that workers became concerned for their own safety and compelled their unions to petition OSHA for help. OSHA adopted requirements closely following CDC guidelines for preventing the transmission of HIV and hepatitis B virus and other blood-borne diseases.[25]

This is not to say that dental offices were unsanitary. The science of disinfection and sterilization had been in place since 1881, ever since Robert Koch researched the disinfecting properties of steam and hot air. By the turn of the century, dentists knew enough to wash their hands between patients and boil their instruments.[26] However, since orthodontists seldom do invasive procedures, before the early '80s the use of cold disinfection techniques and ungloved hands had been the standard of care. As late as 1981, only 24% of 431 oral surgeons surveyed used gloves with all patients.[27]

By the mid-80s, most state boards had adopted regulations based on CDC infection-control procedures (renamed *universal precautions* in 1988). Foremost was the wearing of protective clothing by dental health workers (gloves, gowns, masks, and eyewear). Chemical disinfectants had to be replaced with heat-sterilizing techniques (autoclaves).[28] Of course, this necessitated a special area to set them up, plus additional personnel and instruments to maintain the cycle.

Other safeguards included the use of disposable items where possible, special handling of contaminated waste (no longer could you hand a child his or her extracted tooth!), and offering auxiliaries free immunizations against hepatitis B.[29] Special provision had to be made for disposal of "sharps (needles, scalpels, etc.)." Whereas orthodontists seldom gave injections, used archwires were placed in the same category as needles and had to be embedded in rigid, leak- and puncture-resistant containers else they infected an innocent bystander. Wire cages began to appear around Dumpsters to prevent theft of needles.

Safety in the workplace mandated by OSHA's Hazard Communication Standard of August 1984 necessitated eyewash stations, labeling of chemicals, maintaining a file of material safety data sheets, posting of EXIT signs, purchase of a medical emergency kit, and a written hazard communication plan, an exposure control plan, and a hazardous waste management plan.[30]

Dentists were overwhelmed with what to them was a clear case of legislative overkill. Bellavia stated in 1992 that the additional supplies could add $50 to $100 to the cost of each new patient and require an average staff time of perhaps 3 minutes per patient.[31] Typical was the reaction of Harry H. "Skip" Lawrence, a Sacramento, California, dentist.

> I recently viewed an OSHA video tape on recommended sterilization techniques. It was absolutely unbelievable. It would require 20 minutes of downtime to completely spray down and sterilize the operatory after each patient. I can't believe anyone will ever follow those recommendations to the letter.[32]

Thomas S. McLellan, chairman of the Michigan Dental Association Special Committee on Health and Hazard Regulations, criticizes the dental profession for taking a "reactive," rather than a "proactive," position when threatened with new government activity. "Had the health care industry taken a serious attitude and adopted industry-wide standards for the protection of workers against blood-borne pathogens, the implementation of another unwelcome regulation might have been prevented."[33]

Managed Care

By the late 1960s, the growth of prepaid dental programs had reached enormous proportions, to the extent that the orthodontic specialty was not prepared to deal with it. "Confusion, apprehension, concern, lack of interest, rebellion, apathy, bewilderment might well be some of the terms with which to define the feelings of orthodontists across the country with respect to prepaid dental programs.... The AAO central office ... have been endeavoring to keep abreast of the mountain of reports, proposals, and legislation that relate to us," reported AAO executive secretary James E. Brophy during a meeting in Boston in October 1966.[34]

Definitions. Gone were the days of pure *fee-for-service*, wherein all patients simply paid the bill out-of-pocket. *Indemnity insurance* is another way to make treatment more affordable, yet allow doctors to maintain their standard fees. Here the patient is reimbursed for a loss (the doctor's bill) just as he or she would be reimbursed under a life or a homeowner's policy. *Assigned payments* are made directly to the doctor, but the doctor can refuse to accept *assignment*. After initial resistance, by 1996 more than 82% of orthodontists were accepting assigned benefits.[35] The patients have their choice of doctor but, of course, they must pay higher out-of-pocket costs. In line with their efforts to contain health-care costs, insurance people argue that, since doctors are reimbursed for every service performed, traditional insurance provides a greater incentive for expensive treatment.[36]

At the other end of the spectrum is capitation, administered by a *health maintenance organization* (HMO). In this type of plan, the doctor is paid an agreed-upon monthly fee for each person enrolled in the plan regardless of whether participants use the doctor's service. Since the doctor must be concerned that the cost of treating those patients does not exceed the capitation payments plus patient fees, he or she becomes, in a sense, an insurer. The patient may see only a participating doctor and, under orthodontic plans, usually pays a reduced fee for the treatment. The orthodontist, in turn, agrees to treat any patient who so requests (and needs) it. Furthermore, the doctor may be financially penalized for referring the patient to another specialist (if, for example, an orthodontist refers the patient to an oral surgeon for the extraction of wisdom teeth), and receives no more money if costs exceed the capitation payments. Under the capitation system, health care costs are said to be *contained*, because the practitioner will think twice before ordering expensive tests, etc. Also, prevention is encouraged. This last point may well apply to medicine and general dentistry, but malocclusion is generally difficult to prevent.

The AAO, at its 1982 annual session, advanced its objections to capitation programs:

1. They do not give the patient freedom of choice.
2. They do not offer the best methods of peer review or quality assurance.
3. They limit the use of orthodontists.
4. They place the orthodontist at financial risk.[37]

Between the two extremes of fee-for-service and HMOs are *preferred provider organizations* (PPOs). The doctors, or *providers*, participating in these plans are "preferred" by the insurance carrier, or *third party*, because they have agreed to discount their normal fees. In return for this discount, the carrier includes the names of participating orthodontists on lists given to member patients. In promoting the plan to practitioners, the insurance company offers the bait of additional patients to fill the orthodontist's empty chairs. This works fine until the doctor finds that his or her fee-for-service patients are subsidizing the PPO patients.

Fees offered to PPO providers were often little more than 50% of prevailing fees. In 1983, when the average fee on the West Coast was $2,600, orthodontists who had signed up with Blue Cross of California could charge member patients only $1,400. Arthur A. Dugoni, orthodontist and at the time Dean of the University of the Pacific School of Dentistry, called it "an insult to the orthodontic profession, similar to asking a contractor to build a house for less than his costs. . . ." and predicted that, if such organizations were allowed to continue unchecked, they would "shatter the very foundations of our health delivery system." He also urged the PCSO to "inform its members so that they will make an informed decision before they jump in."[38]

Both HMO and PPO plans are features of *managed care*. Although managed care was new to dentistry, its roots in medicine reached back over 100 years (see Table I). Its original intent was to guarantee health care to enrollees and to foster preventive medicine. Today, according to AAO public relations literature, the concept has more to do with managing costs than with managing care. These plans rely on the volume discount principle. By selling a larger volume of a *product* (the term used by insurance companies), it is possible to charge less for each unit and still realize a profit. While this principle may work for discount houses, it does not apply to health care because the doctor can see only so many patients in a day.

Table I

Historical Highlights of Managed Care

1851	1st private prepaid health plan in US—French Mutual Benevolent Society, San Francisco
1880s	Mandatory sickness insurance (later called "health insurance") coverage in Germany—Otto von Bismarck
1908-13	Raymond G Taylor, MD—prepayment arrangement to provide health services to 10,000 workers building liberty ships
1916	Failure of 1st attempt to introduce universal health insurance in the US
1924	1st California hospital-based Blue Cross-like plan—Golden State Hospital Benefit Fund, Los Angeles
1929	1st California prepaid medical group practice—Ross-Loos Medical Group, with Los Angeles water and power depts. In 1934, Drs Ross and Loos were expelled from LA Medical Society
1930	Sidney Garfield, MD—prepaid health plan for workers on Colorado River Aqueduct (later, Hoover and Grand Coulee dams)—roots of Kaiser Permanente Health Plan
1932	American Medical Assn issued statement strongly opposing prepaid medical care, leading to the founding of Blue Cross
1932–33	Most extensive health insurance scandal in American history, due to rapid expansion in HMO-like hospital and health association growth (California)

Mid-30s	Benjamin Franklin Life Assurance Co and Pacific Employers Ins Co experimented with what today would be called exclusive provider arrangements for health benefits (declared illegal)
1937	1st urban precursor of HMOs—Group Health Assn of Washington, DC—brainchild of Home Owner's Loan Corp
1939	1st statewide Blue Shield Plan—California Physicians Service, formed by California Medical Association
1942	Kaiser expands prepayment role to cover workers building liberty ships
1947	Taft-Hartley Labor Management and Relations Act allowed employers to create health benefits and other schemes to supplement workers' income
1956	1st capitated health plan devoted to children's dental care (Harbor City, Calif)
1971	Pres Nixon's health message to Congress led to extensive growth of HMOs
1975	Knox-Keene Act recognized that health care plans were proliferating in California and that oversight was necessary. Sought to ensure that California residents were guaranteed quality health care from registered health plans

Table I source - Sources: Peter Grant, "History of the California Health System," *California Hospitals* 3, 4, and 5 (1989–1991).
Thomas R. Mayer and Gloria G. Mayer, "Occasional Notes. HMOs: Origin and Development," *New England J Med* 312 (28 Feb. 1985):590–594.
Julian Singer, "History of Managed Care Dentistry," lecture delivered at UCLA, June 9, 1997.

Difficulties. Although medical costs—at least until recently—had been skyrocketing, dental care in 1996 was less expensive than it had been 25 years ago (in constant dollars).[39] In the orthodontic specialty, it cost the typical American worker in 1952 about 432 hours of labor to purchase treatment for a child. In 1997, the parent needed to work only 279 hours for the same treatment. Compare that with the cost of a single-family home which in 1952 took 6,528 hours of work vs 10,480 hours then.[40]

The additional paper work brought its own set of problems. If the forms were not filled out correctly, payments would be delayed. If payments were late in coming to indemnity patients, they would complain not to the carrier, but to the orthodontic office, because it was "there." Additional personnel were needed and the term *insurance girl* came into the lexicon. What's more, orthodontists resented having their treatment plans questioned by nonprofessionals.

Eligibility requirements were another source of friction—often between colleagues. An orthodontic consultant, himself board certified, sent a caustic

31

letter to a Washington provider, rebuking him for failing to send records on one of the panel's patients and stating in part, "It is my hope that you will be most comfortable when you advise the H—— family that they will not be able to receive coverage . . . [since] . . . you refuse to send orthodontic records." A copy was sent to the patient's parents. Donald M. Wright of the Washington State Association of Orthodontists, called it "a flagrant and regrettable violation of the orthodontist's relationship with the family. . . "[41]

To correct these conflicts, as well as promote the highest standards of excellence in orthodontic treatment, the AAO at its 1974 annual meeting adopted a resolution concerning prepayment procedures. One of these was that the third party should reimburse the patient directly as fees are incurred. Payment should not be premised according to accomplishment of arbitrary phases or procedural steps of treatment, nor on frequency of appointments. Further, the third party must allow the patients their traditional right to the free selection of an orthodontist—not by the publication of lists of participating practitioners.[42]

Opponents of free choice argued that this system actually results in inferior care at excessive cost because (1) the individual is not in a position to judge competence, since the choice is usually based upon the reports of friends, neighbors, or relatives with respect to fees and personality traits, (2) the doctor's popularity is not a measure of his or her ability, and (3) fee-for-service emphasizes curative rather than preventive care. What's more, free choice encourages "shopping around," something doctors themselves oppose.[43]

The "fight-'em-or-join-'em" dilemma. Many orthodontists thought that signing up with a large insurance company would alleviate the collection problem, but it only transferred the problem to an invisible entity. In a letter to CHAMPUS (Civilian Health and Medical Program of the Uniformed Services) from the California State Society of Orthodontists (CSSO), President Donald R. Poulton complained that payments and claim handling had fallen as much as 6 months behind in some cases and that the abrupt cessation of the quarterly billing system for patients in the middle of treatment might well be grounds for a breach of contract suit.[44] Nor was dealing with governmental agencies a guarantee of payment. In 1971, when Alameda County ran out of funds, they simply abandoned payment on a number of Crippled Children's Services cases that had already been started.[45]

Starting in the late 1970s, orthodontists who had signed up with Maxicare, one of the largest HMOs, were getting $1,000 as the treatment fee in addition to their monthly capitation. If the utilization rate did not become too high, it was possible for a participating office to realize approximately $2,500 for each case treated (over a period of two years), about the prevailing fee at the time. However, Maxicare expanded too rapidly and in

1989 was forced into bankruptcy, leaving participating orthodontists high and dry.[46]

Despite leaders' urgings to use caution in entering into capitation contracts, many practitioners succumbed to economic pressures. In 1976, Donald A. Rudee, CSSO President, was being realistic when he said, "The conscientious orthodontist can only hold out so long, as he sees patients taken away from his office and into that of his undercutting neighbor." No one knew this better than third-party recruiters. "The advocates of competitive bidding in the marketplace did not need advanced degrees in psychology to know that survival, fear, and greed would capture the orthodontist as it would any other segment. There will always be those who would take a capitation contract and would make a profit treating for $1,000 a case."[47]

The orthodontist who had chosen to practice in a town dominated by one employer also found himself caught between the proverbial rock and a hard place. If the employer signed up for managed care and the majority of patients were covered by that plan, the orthodontist had three options: accept a mixed practice, get along without insurance patients, or leave town.[48]

One might ask, "Look at the gains made in the past by labor groups and minorities. Why couldn't orthodontists stand united against insurance companies and others trying to whittle them down?" For one thing, explained Rocky Mountain Society of Orthodontists president Fred J. Wuthrich, minorities had "many dedicated individuals willing to work long hours, with much sacrifice, in order to gain what they considered rightfully theirs. . . . The difference in the two groups is that the first was hungry, and the second [the orthodontists] is not."[49] Besides, cautioned John Miles, AAO attorney, "there's little a professional association of competing providers can do or say about PPOs without risking antitrust liability. . . . Any effort by two or more orthodontists to boycott, restrain, or take any illegal action to restrain a PPO from competing successfully is against the law."[50] Moreover, "the AAO cannot establish or mandate . . . uniform prices or fee would be price fixing."[51]

A precedent for this was set in 1986 when the US Supreme Court upheld the findings of an antitrust violation involving a "union" of Indiana dentists in pursuing a policy of resisting insurer requests for radiographs. The court held that labor's exemption from antitrust laws applies only to nonsupervisory employees bargaining collectively with their employers.[52]

However, there was a perfectly legal way for dentistry to have dealt with managed care, by following medicine's example: independent practice (or physicians') associations (IPAs). These are practitioner-owned associations that serve as their organized negotiating channels in dealing with HMOs and insurance companies. Why several attempts to organize them in dentistry failed may be due to the fact that dentists are characteristically solo practitioners, while physicians tend to cluster into groups working in hospital settings.[53]

Just as insurance companies were able to take advantage of economic pressures to obtain contracts for low-fee dental services, so were labor unions able to set up contracts and, in many cases, closed-panel clinics for package deals. These deals involved large segments of the dental population.[54] In some cases, unions did not hesitate to flaunt their power. In his presidential message, Lloyd L. Cottingham of the PCSO told members that ". . . trust fund officers have told us that they could open a 'closed shop,' hire our members, and tell your society to go to ——. As an association of professional men, we do not have a czar's jurisdiction over our members."[55]

Economic Forces

Despite a 117% increase in the Consumer Price Index (CPI) between 1970 and 1980, orthodontists' income rose only 37%. Also, their fees lagged somewhat at 105%. However, the major factor in their loss of earning power was a drop in case starts of 33%.[56] Whether or not it was intended that way, Senator Orrin Hatch (R.-Utah) praised dentistry's ability to keep its fees 16% below the change in the CPI between 1972 and 1982, by saying on the floor of Congress that "dentistry's record of cost restraint is, in my opinion, an impressive one . . . ."[57] Furthermore, three recessions occurring close together during this period (early 1976, early '80, and '81–82)[58] kept fees from rising, but orthodontists were hesitant about readjusting them during recoveries because of increasing competition.

In a lagging economy one would expect jobseekers to proliferate, but such was not the case with office help. It was becoming harder and harder to find RDAs to help chairside, and staff turnover plagued many offices. One of the reasons was that other industries, especially large companies, were offering important fringe benefits such as health insurance. Another was the increasing number and complexity of skills required.[59] Results of a 1985 survey by the AAO suggested that auxiliaries had a desire for more continuing education. Other complaints included the frustration of working with unmotivated patients and, of course, low pay.[60] Doctors who finally brought their benefits into line saw their costs mount.

Consumerism

After World War II new interest arose in consumer protection. It gained additional momentum after 1965 with Ralph Nader's *Unsafe at Any Speed*. The public responded by demanding investigation of not only cars, but other products, business practices, and advertising. Consumerism gave rise to boycotts, lawsuits and, finally, the passage of laws affecting all aspects of the marketplace.[61]

One of the first to involve dentistry was the Truth in Lending Act (1965), requiring fee disclosure in contracts. Other laws imposed controls on office sanitation, workplace safety, employee relations, and accommodation of the handicapped. And more controls meant more overhead. Meanwhile consumer advocates, using the power of television, urged the public to be better informed, demand better service, and obtain more value for their dollar.

Opportunism

Another force that could be classed as economic will be labeled, for the purpose of this account, opportunism. To be sure, *opportunism* is what allowed third-party organizations to take advantage of dentists' "unbusyness."

Litigation. The most devastating form of opportunism is litigation. Until the 1980s, lawsuits against orthodontists were rare. Possibly the main reason for this was the fact that most treatment results were at least satisfactory in the eyes of the patient. A second reason was that the extended period of treatment gave the parties an opportunity to develop a friendly relationship; it is unusual for people to sue friends. Third, poor results are often due to failure of patient cooperation (as long as the patient and/or parents are aware of this). Finally, the proportion of adult patients—who are less tolerant of discomfort and whose tissues are less forgiving—was low.

Since orthodontics often causes extensive changes in the occlusion, there is more likelihood of temporomandibular joint (TMJ) problems, which could trigger pain, spasm, or joint sounds. Some of these conditions may have been present subclinically. With young women—the group most likely to manifest such problems—making up the largest group of adults undergoing orthodontic treatment, it is readily seen how the increasing prevalence of "TMJ" (as the public usually calls it) can add to the orthodontist's vulnerability.[62]

Burakoff and Demby, in a symposium on quality assurance, cited other reasons for the growing prevalence of lawsuits: "higher expectations of professional performance, impersonality of the health care system, a breakdown in professional screening and discipline (due to the growth in the number of practitioners), and ambitious malpractice lawyers."[63] In addition, there is a lack of penalties for frivolous lawsuits.

Typical of the TMJ brouhaha was the suit brought against the PCSO in 1975 (*Kean vs PCSO*) for $200,000 plus punitive damages for "damages resulting from injuries sustained through the negligent conduct and malpractice" of one of its members. The Central Section of the society argued that "there is no standard and reliable method known for preventing the temporomandibular joint syndrome . . . nor was it a matter of instruction in dental schools." The case was finally settled for $4,000.[64]

Not so fortunate was an orthodontist in southeastern Michigan (*Brimm vs* ——-) who in 1987 was embroiled in the largest suit in orthodontic history (seeking $1 million). As before, the complaint involved the TMJ. Even though an expert witness testified that the orthodontist had obtained a superior result that could have been used as a display case for specialty board certification[65] and, even though no scientific evidence was presented by the plaintiff, the defendant was forced to settle out of court for $800,000[66] causing concern that a dangerous precedent had been set whereby scientific controversies could be settled in a court of law rather than the usual professional channels.[67]

By 1984, California was producing 4000 attorneys a year. Analysts expected an attorney population of a million in the state by 1990.[68] Not only has the frequency of litigation against orthodontists risen since 1980, but so have liability insurance rates. In southern Florida, for example, a solo orthodontist might have paid as much as $15,000 a year for malpractice protection.[69] To defend against these lawsuits, a whole new "subspecialty" of practice had arisen: the orthodontist with a law degree.

Other forms of opportunism. Despite AAO representation on the Joint Commisssion Accreditation of Dental Laboratories, the labs had a new approach. Now their emphasis was on removables and specialized laboratories to make them. *The Newsletter of Modern Prosthetic Techniques* stated bluntly, "The general practitioner works harder, longer, and for less money than the orthodontist. As a consequence, general practitioners are starting to turn to orthodontics." Adding that the amount of tooth repair is dropping, one way to make up for it is for the GP to offer minor tooth movement. There should be no problem—so said the labs—finding patients from among the 40 million estimated malocclusions in the United States. And to assist the general dentist in handling this bonanza, the newsletter suggested that the dental laboratories set up their own orthodontic departments.[70]

Taking advantage of the recently instituted continuing education requirement and the desire for GPs to get on the "gravy train," certain lecturers began offering short orthodontic courses. These courses were derisively called "motel courses" or "tailgate courses" by the establishment and usually had the following characteristics:

1. They were given by self-styled gurus whose experience was outside the traditional university setting.
2. They touted some particular technique.
3. The appliance was relatively simple.
4. The aspect of making money was frequently emphasized.
5. A cookbook approach was used.
6. Scientific evidence, if any, did not include long-term studies.

Group Practice

The idea of group practice, that is, the practicing together of two or more doctors as one entity, was not a new concept in orthodontics, and certainly not in dentistry. Painless Parker evolved the concept back in 1893, when he realized that a lone, single-handed dentist could not provide good dentistry at an economical cost.[71] The McCoy brothers were orthodontics' first model group practice in the 1920s (see above, under Harbinger of the Future). The first three-man orthodontic group on the West Coast had been operating in Portland, Oregon, since 1955 (telephone interview with Guy A. Woods, January 1996).

Now, with the National Housing Act encouraging loans to groups for construction and the Knox-Keene Act permitting dentists to incorporate, group practices were formed with a vengeance. Even a solo dentist could hire one associate and call the entity a "group." Groups were to have both positive and negative effects on the orthodontic specialty.

In addition to legal incentives, there were other reasons for GPs to meld. The most obvious was economies of scale. Space, equipment, supplies, and personnel could be shared. Greater choice could now be offered the patient, both in terms of doctors and, by staggering personnel shifts, in terms of appointment times. More evening and Saturday hours became available.

Having one's colleagues at hand gave group members the benefit of wider knowledge and here, too, was built-in peer review. Vacations and emergency coverage were more easily arranged. Senior members could retire without abruptly "closing shop." By the same token, the corporate practice would have perpetuity.

But what affected orthodontists most keenly was the concept of multispecialties. Dentists disliked having patients leave their offices to see specialists. Kickbacks were either illegal or unethical, so one way to share in the patient's total care was to have all the specialties "under one roof." In addition, patients had the comfort of knowing that all their dental needs could be taken care of in familiar surroundings.

Usually the specialists attended only on a part-time basis; therefore, they could be associated with more than one group. They might even have private practices of their own. The group would hire, or become partners with, a pediatric dentist, an oral surgeon, a periodontist—and an orthodontist. Thus, an orthodontist recently out of school could have an income while building his or her own practice. Everyone was pleased with this arrangement except the neighborhood orthodontist to whom that office formerly referred.

Discount dentistry. From group practice the next logical step in the commercialization of dental care was what could best be called "discount" dentistry. Under this heading are included department store dentistry, retail dentistry, and corporate dentistry. Just as there can be overlapping between these entities, so has the term, "clinics," been applied across the board to them by organized dentistry. Their common denominators were high volume, low fee, extensive use of registered dental assistants (RDAs), dentists-for-hire (including orthodontists), and heavy advertising.

The usual procedure wherein multiple locations were involved was to break down the staff into teams, each team servicing a different clinic each day (since a given clinic did not necessarily operate full-time). For economy's sake, instruments and supplies were transported by the staff from location to location. Each clinic had its own orthodontist, although he or she could attend more than one clinic.

Even though latter-day clinics shared some traits with those of the 1940s and '50s, they were not descendants. The early clinics did not feature extended-duty auxiliaries, they did not advertise to any great extent, and they were not primarily general dentistry facilities with "ortho" as an afterthought, as are the clinics of today.

Department store dentistry originally referred to those dental facilities located in a retail department store or drug store. Later, it applied more to the philosophy of approaching the public. Patterned after a consumer-oriented business, it also had certain particular practice characteristics, such as high visibility, easy access, use of extensive advertising, reduced fees, extensive use of auxiliaries, and availability of specialty services. Other distinguishing features included extended hours, no appointments necessary, all work done on the premises (most completed the same day), care of a given patient by multiple dentists, high volume, salaried dentists, and high personnel turnover.[72]

The first modern department store dental center in the United States was opened in a Sears department store in El Monte, California, in 1976.[73] It was followed soon afterward by a Hempstead, New York, dentist (Allan Gutstein) who was quick to take advantage of the 1977 Supreme Court ruling on advertising. Orthodontics was offered in many of the facilities. A sampling of orthodontic fees in 1977 from three of the clinics reveals a range of $800 to $1,000 per case, compared with private fees of $1,187 to $1,708.[74] By July 1981, 18 department stores and 3 drug store chains had installed 63 retail store dental facilities in 14 states and the District of Columbia.[75]

Retail dentistry. Most department store dental centers have disappeared and have been replaced with retail, or "store-front," dental offices where they are afforded a high degree of visibility in today's minimalls. However, many conventional dentists also find it advantageous to locate in minimalls, as opposed to professional buildings.

Corporate dentistry. One does not need a boardroom and a penthouse suite to incorporate. A dentist with one operatory can become a corporation, as long as he or she fulfills the legal requirements. Corporate dentistry, at the other extreme, involves large-scale operations with more than 20 chairs, frequently in multiple locations. Facilities of such magnitude require large capital outlays. Thus it was only natural that Knox-Keene–licensed dental plans, already involved with PPOs and HMOs, would take a step further and open their own clinics, or "staff model offices." Among the pioneers of this concept were Consumer Health (later, Newport Dental Plan), Safeguard Health Plans, and SmileCare Dental.[76] Unions also backed clinics indirectly by contracting with individual dentists to service their members and dependents.

Another category of dental entrepreneur was the old credit dentist, moving out of the era of "plates." R.F. Beauchamp was the first to open multiple offices, using the name Dr Beauchamp/Western Dental Centers (telephone interview with Philip Megdal, July 1995).

Individual dentists or dental groups with sufficient backing, business acumen, and the foresight to see that prepaid dentistry was the wave of the future, were able to get on the bandwagon before the big health plans took over. One of the first—and most successful—of these was Howard M. Stein. Opening an office in West Covina, California, in 1967, Stein parlayed his practice into two clinics (the other in Bellflower) boasting some 90 chairs. He achieved this with the help of the Henry J. Kaiser steelworkers and other unions.

Orthodontic services were added in the early 1970s. Stein's fees were generally lower than private practitioners, of course, but not by much. "When they were charging $2700 for a 2-year, full-banded case, I was probably charging $2200 or 2300 [including records and retainers]," said Stein in a telephone interview in December 1995. "I remember some guys cut fees down to $1800, with SmileCare doing it at $1200. This was now in the early '80s."

Was money the chief motivation of these dental empire-builders, who not only took great risks, but flew in the face of organized dentistry? Stein says, "From the time I was in dental school, I always envisioned being able to deliver dentistry at reasonable fees, on a no-frills basis, and reaching people who never got to dental offices, but who could afford to come to mine."

In addition to profitability, clinic owners' major problems were quality control, staff turnover, and standardization—trying to get orthodontic "prima donnas" to use uniform appliances and procedures. Stein admits, "We had constant problems with quality control. If you had a bad dentist, you had to find out and get rid of him. [But] I never had a real problem with ortho."

Ronald T. Aiello, orthodontic manager for a union plan in the 1970s, pointed out via telephone interview in October 1995, that competence is a highly individual matter:

> I can cite you people who were presidents of dental societies, in private practice, who had their . . . assistants working and they weren't even there. . . . The ones who chose this mode of practice [clinics] were not necessarily less competent. It was more due to wanting to avoid, or not being capable of, dealing with the business aspects of private practice.

However, he did allow that doctor turnover had a negative effect on treatment.

"Some of the men just wanted to come in, make their per diem, and leave. Usually these people don't stay very long in one place." Reasons for the turnover included doctor's loss of identity, inability to build his or her own practice, and the fast pace. Recent graduates gained experience making a hurried diagnosis and learned how to delegate duties. Older clinicians either adapted or fell by the wayside.

Other challenges included the pressure to finish cases "on time" (meaning in 24 months when monthly payments ran out), conforming to office protocol (such as getting along without your favorite pliers or forgoing an appliance that would have triggered a lab bill), or making the best of untrained RDAs (due to their scarcity). Also, many foreign dentists, who were unlicensed in the United States and were finding work as chairside assistants, had language difficulties.

Leonard D. Birnkrant, who worked as a temporary orthodontist in the office of Dr ——-, recalled in a telephone interview with the author in July 1995: "They asked me if I could spend a couple of days there. I'm looking at this work. There are no records. I can't figure out what the guy's trying to do. The next day I looked at some more cases. They were so bad that I had to go home and take a shower."

So much, then, for insiders' comments. What did impartial reviewers have to say about quality of care? Lawrence L. Furstman, who inspected orthodontic offices for prepaid plans, stated in a December 1987 telephonic interview, "I've been in offices where they have 10 or 12 chairs, with a girl at each chair. The doctor does nothing but look in each patient's mouth with a tongue blade, make a note in the chart, and that's it. I don't think that's right."

To ensure quality care, the Knox-Keene Act of 1975 mandates that the California Department of Corporations (DOC) conduct periodic on-site surveys of health-plan delivery systems. The review is all-encompassing and includes an evaluation of the overall facility, equipment, personnel, patient access, infection control, facility forms, radiological safety, emergency preparedness, documentation, and treatment outcome.[76]

Dr ——- has been conducting such inspections since 1987. In addition, he has reviewed private offices for a PPO since 1982. He has found that the majority of problems associated with managed care were those that are not readily apparent to the patient, adding in a July 1995 phone interview, "What happens with these plans is that they have beautiful facilities, good sterilization, a lot of people working there, but they don't take too many records. When I go out, I like to review 20 completed cases. I rarely get that. If I get two or three, I'm lucky." One harried orthodontic director told the reviewer, "I'm charging $775 for a case and you expect me to take records on these people?"

Dr —— found that, based on the few final records he did see, results in clinic facilities were generally unsatisfactory. Yet many of the individual (nonclinic) PPO providers—some of them board-certified—were no better. In rebuttal to managed-care providers' oft-made claim, he said, "It's true that a lot of people are now getting orthodontic care who would never have gotten it before, but I'm not sure you could call it good care." Is it possible for good orthodontics to be done in a clinic environment? "There's a handful of offices doing this kind of mass orthodontics, that do very acceptable work . . . but the rest I just have no use for. . . . You have to have somebody in charge who is motivated to do good work."

FORCES WITHIN ORTHODONTICS

There is a word in the medical vocabulary, *iatrogenic*, that means "any adverse condition in a patient resulting from treatment by a physician or surgeon."[77] Applying a liberal interpretation to this term, the writer will attempt to show that many of the ills besetting the specialty of orthodontics during the period of decline were iatrogenic.

Technology

Even technology had its adverse effects. In the early 1950s, when the California State Dental Association assessed its members to promote statewide fluoridation, the *San Francisco Examiner* editorialized: "Take your hats off to a group of professional people who would assess themselves $18 a year to put themselves out of business." (According to Raymond M. Curtner during a telephone interview in December 1994.) However, the initial humor soon wore off as thousands of practitioners found themselves with gaps in their appointment books. To fill these gaps, many general practitioners added orthodontics to their services.

Again, technology made it easier for this to happen. In the late 1950s preformed bands eliminated both the skill required to "pinch" and solder bands, and the time needed to "strap up" a case. Then, in the early '70s, bonded brackets not only cut this time further but appreciably reduced band inventory requirements. The next logical step in eliminating the term "metal mouth" was to replace the metal bracket with a tooth-colored material such as plastic (early '70s) or ceramic (late '80s). Another approach—much more difficult for the operator—was lingual brackets ("invisible braces"), perfected in the late '70s. Preformed archwires and a programmed set of brackets called the "straight wire" appliance nearly took the nickname "wirebender" out of the vocabulary. Another breakthrough, "memory" or "superelastic" wire, dramatically reduced the time needed to "level" the teeth. Unfortunately for the establishment, bonded brackets and preadjusted appliances also made orthodontics more attractive to GPs and pediatric dentists.

In 1970, Rolf Fränkel, an East German orthodontist, introduced his function regulator (FR) for the orthopedic correction of Class II malocclusions. It was embraced by general practitioners because it required only a set of impressions and a wax bite. It did not require the large inventory of bands and instruments, and it eliminated the need to extract teeth.[78] These innovations, along with auxiliaries' expanded duties, made the treatment of malocclusions increasingly attractive to the GP, while orthodontic supply houses were only too happy to provide the wherewithal.

Bonded brackets, recycled bands and brackets, and answering machines were about the only technological advances that resulted in savings. Computerizing an office could run into the tens of thousands. Copy machines, fax machines, and hi-tech telephones added their costs. Digital photography and radiography were yet to come.

Recycling became a very controversial topic. There was something repugnant about the idea of placing in your patient's mouth something that had spent months in someone else's. On the other hand, when you take your family to Applebee's for dinner, do you expect to find spanking-new silverware on your table? In the hospital, do you know how many times your catheter has been in someone else's vein? Should you get informed consent before strapping up a patient in secondhand hardware?

In 1976, Romanian-born Claude G. Matasa, a chemical engineer, was convinced that there was a place for the reconditioning of orthodontic brackets. All he had to do was to figure out how to turn out a product that was unmarred, uncontaminated, and irreproachable; convince orthodontists it would be to their advantage to use them; get the stamp of approval from product-safety agencies; make a profit; and weather the storm of protests that was sure to come from bracket manufacturers.

These took the form of attempts to frighten the public away from accepting recycled brackets via a *Fight Back* segment on NBC-TV to outright lawsuits. Finally Matasa, now heading a company called Ortho-Cycle, was exonerated when AAO president Donald Poulton deemed them "safe and effective." Furthermore, Ortho-Cycle was given a CE mark by the prestigious Scandinavian Institute of Dental Materials. Along the way, Ortho-Cycle has not only saved money for orthodontists, but has improved the environment by reducing the amount of harmful chemicals (discarded brackets) being dumped into our groundwater, and helped legitimize the overall concept of medical and dental recycling.

Graduate Glut

If the output of new graduates had been keyed to the decline in the patient pool, then the patients-per-orthodontist ratio might have remained favorable. But by 1970, 350 fledgling orthodontists were completing their training each year, according to Paul R. Reid, president of the Middle Atlantic Society of Orthodontists. In only 11 years, from 1964 to 1975, AAO membership more than doubled (from 3,313 to 8,606). Even so, the leadership still held out the hope that a resurgence of orthodontic demand was on the horizon. Said Reid, "It is estimated by 1970, 15 million children on some form of public assistance will be eligible for free treatment. Add to this the large number of patients who will come under private prepaid programs, and it is apparent to anyone that the ratio between need and demand will change considerably."[79]

Attitude Toward Public

Initially, lack of competition kept fees high and hours inconvenient. A father would joke, "My kids' braces paid for Dr Smith's boat." There were no evening hours; few offices opened Saturdays. There were justifiable reasons for office scheduling policies, but parents disliked taking their children out of school. More and more mothers were entering the work force, leaving Junior without transportation.

As the doctor's staff grew, he or she spent more time managing and less time at the chair. This became especially true after new laws gave chairside assistants extended duties and technology cut treatment corners. Harvey M. Spears, 1972 president of the PCSO, admitted, "We have also tended to treat patients as 'cases' rather than human beings. . . . There no longer is the close personal contact . . ."[80] Thirteen years later, the same complaint was voiced by Harry L. Dougherty, chairman of the University of Southern California orthodontic department. "In the busy practice of today, minimum time is devoted to taking a history, listening to the patient's needs and concerns, and fully explaining the treatment outcome and limitations . . . . [orthodontists] have delegated the examination and consultation procedure to ancillary personnel."[81]

Sometimes idealism got in the way. Many were reluctant to do less than a full corrective job, when patients desired only limited correction.[82]

Intradental Relations

Ever since specialists broke away from mainstream dentists, relations had been strained. Now, with unbusyness affecting both groups, the strain became more acute. The old problems of excluding nonspecialists from orthodontic associations, restricting attendance at postgraduate courses, and discouraging AAO members from participating in short courses unless sponsored by universities or local orthodontic societies were still in evidence.

When it came to getting AAO members to teach undergraduate students, each side accused the other of noncooperation. Orthodontists accused dental school administrators of failing to provide the necessary time in the curriculum; yet, when students asked, "Why no orthodontics?" they were told that orthodontists are not willing to "give up their tricks of the trade."[83]

In his first message as PCSO president, Warren A. Kitchen called intradental relations "the most pertinent problem that our society and our specialty faces at this time." Following a meeting between officers of the PCSO and CDA, he reported that "we are not talking to each other enough and the orthodontists appeared greedy, self-interest-seeking in the eyes of our colleagues."[84]

Typical of the infighting was the reaction of the Maine State Orthodontic Society (MSOS) to an ad placed by a general dentist for orthodontic care. The MSOS responded with major radio and newspaper announcements questioning the ability of GPs to provide orthodontic service equal to that of orthodontists. Taking keen offense, the Academy of General Dentistry (AGD) called their response "a violation of the spirit of Section 8 of the

American Dental Association's Principles of Ethics. . . ." and that the MSOS was "commenting disparingly [sic], without justification, about all of the family dentists . . ."[85]

In an effort to promote a better understanding of the need for specialty education, as well as set up guidelines for the teaching of undergraduate orthodontics, the respective councils on education of the ADA and AAO held a series of conferences. The outcome of these meetings was a set of guidelines offered in 1976 by the AAO House of Delegates, stating, in essence, that the general dentist should be trained to identify orthodontic problems, treat localized and uncomplicated ones, and realize the necessity for consultation with a specialist.[86]

Complacency

During his or her many years of sacrifice to gain a degree, the doctor-to-be had been told, "Once you get your license, you'll be all set." So that once the typical orthodontist was established, he tended to find other outlets for his free time, such as hobbies or investing. There was no incentive to expand or seek new markets. Most practices did not treat more than 100 to 120 patients at a time, because the specialty was strongly influenced by conscientious leaders who tried to instill a philosophy of high treatment standards and professionalism.[87] Patients' complaints notwithstanding, orthodontic fees did not keep pace with overhead costs and the practitioner's cost of living.[88]

Group practice, which offered savings as well as other benefits, was a rarity among orthodontists. In 1953 Garvin noted that dentistry had scarcely more than explored the possibilities of group practice, while medicine had made much progress in that direction.[89]

Orthodontists were still reluctant to organize dental service plans, which was one way to get out from under the yoke of commercial prepaid plans. A precedent for this type of action was established in 1939, when the California Medical Association formed the California Physicians Service in order to defeat Governor Culbert Olson's proposal for compulsory health insurance.[90] The National Association of Dental Service Plans expected this apathy toward the formation and funding of dental service plans to lead buyers of health care to seek out other less-qualified sources. The next step in this progression might be what Salzmann called "social orthodontics." Under this concept, then prevalent in Europe, the orthodontist is told when and what he may or may not do for his patient. Even as he recognized the threat of prepaid plans, Salzmann saw them as a new source of patient referrals, saying that he expected "a spectacular rise in the demand for orthodontic treatment. . . ."[91]

Closely associated with complacency are the terms *nonparticipation* and *noncohesiveness*. There is a tendency for a satisfied constituency to abrogate its responsibilities to its leaders. "To leave all political responsibility to someone else and live our lives as beneficiaries of the efforts of other men endangers our entire organization," warned Rocky Mountain Society of Orthodontists (RMSO) president Randle J. Gardner. "Erosion from within due to apathy, indifference, and ignorance is as real and threatening as any conceived attack from without."[92] Even more outspoken was President Charles K. Sawyer of the Great Lakes society, when he chided, "The vast majority of our members remain relatively uninformed and essentially unconcerned," and pointed out that "adversaries count heavily on our not being able to solve this dilemma."

He then set forth four reasons for the disunity: The first was that until that time in the history of organized orthodontics, there had been no compelling reasons to unify. Second, with respect to delivery systems, the bulk of the membership didn't know enough or care enough to have an opinion. The solution to that problem, of course, lay in educating the membership. The third reason for disunity was the fact that "the same old crowd" often governs from a cloistered position, turning off a significant number of members. Correcting this would require reorganization at all levels to open up lines of communication, give better representation to individual members, and make way for stronger, more articulate leaders. The final reason was the independent nature of the dental species—a major reason for becoming a dentist in the first place. Sawyer admitted that "although this relinquishing of individual thought and action may be the most difficult, I am confident that . . . our membership will respond."[93]

CHAPTER V

Reaction (1968–

BY EDUCATORS

As late as 1974, the question of how many new orthodontists should be trained annually had not been answered. Robert L. Williams, president of the Midwestern Society of Orthodontists and chairman of a special AAO committee studying the problem, estimated that only 150 graduates per year would satisfy the country's orthodontic needs, rather than the then-current 350.[1]

Yet the schools reacted too little and too late. From a high of 352 (first-year postgraduate students) in 1972, the nationwide total dropped less than 20% (to 283) by 1980. For the next 12 years, it remained fairly constant.[2]

Possible reasons for the inertia include, first, institutions do not respond as rapidly as individuals; second, there was the prospect of losing federal funding (which, of course, occurred anyway); and third, being human, administrators and department heads were simply being protective of their turf. As for the funding, by the early '80s, educators' decisions were being made for them: The legislation had expired and the grants had dried up.[3]

BY THE AMERICAN ASSOCIATION OF ORTHODONTISTS

Not since the early '30s when Brodie deemed orthodontics to be "at its lowest ebb," had the specialty been concerned with its very existence. The "baby bust," the performance of treatment by untrained persons, and the incursion of third parties between patient and practitioner were girding the loins of even the most complacent into action. Orthodontics' leaders began putting forth possible solutions. Byron N. Coward, president of the Southwestern Society of Orthodontists (SSO), proposed to (1) pursue a campaign for more and better continuing education, (2) encourage a more equalized distribution of orthodontists, especially in the rural areas, (3) turn out a more realistic number of graduates each year, and (4) encourage members to take a more active part in society affairs.

President H. Curtis Hester of the Middle Atlantic society added four more:

1. Select the profession's leaders more astutely.

2. Let legislators know members' needs while legislation is being written.
3. Learn the language of the bureaucrats in order to communicate with them about "quality assurance" and "levels of competency."
4. Inform the public about the benefits of orthodontic care and that specialists are the best ones to provide it.

With point 4, Coward was in full agreement and, carrying it a step further, called for a vigorous public relations program that would stress the importance and benefits of orthodontics, the need and availability of adult orthodontic treatment, and the importance of securing the services of fully trained orthodontists.[4]

This does not imply that the term "PR" was absent from the vocabulary of organized orthodontics. In the depths of the Depression the ASO (former name of AAO) executive council voted $100 for the purpose of publicizing papers given at annual meetings. A two-man public relations committee was appointed which, in turn, selected a commercial agency to handle the publicity.[5]

During the ensuing years, the committee's activities expanded. In 1968 came a 20-minute, professionally produced slide-tape program entitled "Straight Talk for Straight Teeth," designed for showing at parent groups, schools, and service clubs. The first PR film produced under AAO auspices, "Orthodontics: A Special Kind of Dentistry," was released in 1973 and was deemed "a tremendous success." Also that year, two 30-second TV spot announcements were produced.[6] By 1974, the association had been involved in a wide variety of activities, including an extensive pamphlet program, exhibits, speakers' kits, movies, TV and radio spot announcements, public information, tabletop displays, and continual contact with the news media.[7]

But these efforts paled compared with what was to come. In 1979 the AAO pulled out all the stops with a $2.125-million, major marketing effort. Responding to pressures from members as well as local and state orthodontic societies, the AAO hired the firm of BHN/Doremus to develop programs focused on the use of magazines on a national basis and newspapers and radio on a regional basis. The two-million-dollar-plus price tag was only the first-year budget. While the *advertising* portion of the budget focused on parents of children of orthodontic age, the primary *public relations* effort was on adult orthodontics. Objectives of the program were to (1) expand the market base by increasing the need among those people who affect new-patient decisions, (2) motivate adults to seek care, and (3) give credibility and stature to the AAO. Emphasis was to be placed on long-term health of the mouth (as opposed to cosmetic appearance) and the special qualifications of the specialist in orthodontics.[8]

By far the greatest share of the expenditure ($1.7 million) was allocated to magazine advertising, primarily in *Good Housekeeping, Parent's Magazine, People Weekly,* and *Reader's Digest.* In addition, funds were earmarked to train speakers, hold annual PR seminars in each state and major city, and create a new AAO logo. To finance this campaign, members were assessed $200 and given a 77% dues increase.[9]

But after the second year of assessment, the AAO board of trustees noted that it was unfair to the membership to continue a special assessment year after year when it may have resulted in a substantial loss of members and potential members. Therefore, it was discontinued in the 1982–83 budget.[10]

Results of the marketing program over the first 2 years were encouraging. In little more than 6 months since the program's inception, the AAO office had received over 3,000 letters asking for information on orthodontics.[11] From 1979 to 1981, new patient examinations increased by 10%, new starts increased by 11%, and patients under treatment rose 16%. Moreover, there was a significant change in the ages of treatment. The number of patients under 18 dropped 6%, but those between 18 and 35 rose 27% and the over-35 group grew by 53%.[12]

In 1984 the AAO authorized a yellow-pages program whereby individual members could be listed in a separate section, at their own expense, to indicate that they belonged to the most widely recognized orthodontic organization. The box, showing the AAO logo, bore the inscription, "The orthodontists listed below have completed advanced education required by the American Dental Association to permit announcement as 'Specialist in Orthodontics & Dentofacial Orthopedics.'" The initial cost ranged from $100 to $1100 yearly, depending on the size of the area served.

Not meeting with widespread acceptance, the program was voted down in 1983 by delegates from two of the eight components, with one component divided.[13] Although the listing had positive aspects, opponents of the program pointed out that: (1) It tended to degrade those members declining to "get on the bandwagon," (2) The cost could become prohibitive, as telephone companies continued to carve up their territories, and (3) The public could become confused by nonparticipating members nevertheless listing their AAO membership separately.

BY INDIVIDUAL PRACTITIONERS

Successful orthodontists have always practiced some form of marketing, whether they were conscious of it or not. They were nice to their patients, they developed friendships with the local dentists, and they made themselves known in the community. Even those who were less outgoing did well—there were plenty of patients to go around. Now marketing became as essential as knowing how to fit bands. Those who ignored it had three options: sign up with one or more managed-care plans, go to work for a dental group, or fall by the wayside.

Conscientious practitioners agonized over adopting marketing methods they had long disdained. Now they found that the desire to survive was challenging their disdain. But they need not have compromised their morals, because society was coming to accept such practices and responding more positively to self-promotion done in good taste. The issue was not how ethical was advertising, but rather how its quality could be controlled to enhance the image of orthodontics.[14]

Table II, compiled by *JCO*, lists the marketing activities commonly employed by orthodontists in 1985, about the time most had got over their initial inhibitions about marketing. Although the list includes over 30 strategies, analysis shows that they all more or less fell under four headings:

1. Make yourself known in the community.
2. Make yourself available.
3. Make yourself liked by referral sources.
4. Make the office experience a pleasant one.

Not all orthodontic leaders were enthusiastic about the association's PR program. PCSO president Harvey M. Spears told his constituents that "I personally do not believe the use of TV announcements competing with aspirin or soup would be an effective credit to our specialty. The orthodontist's personal relationship with patient and parents . . . can be the strongest possible source of a favorable public image."[15]

As for advertising in general, San Rafael, California, orthodontist Julian M. Lifschiz had these comments:

> It takes away time and energy from patient care. Doctors are spending more and more time attending meetings to learn how to "sell" dentistry. It is self-escalating. Pretty soon everyone will be at the same point and then someone a little smarter comes up with an idea and then everyone has to do it to stay even.
>
> It is neither professional nor tasteful. The US Supreme Court decision . . . was based on the premise that the public has a right to information. The kind of advertising that is becoming prevalent does not inform, it merely solicits.[16]

Contrasting institutional with individual advertising and at the same time highlighting the absurdity of some of the current tactics, David Turpin editorialized that the AAO was saying, "We are concerned with your health;

we want to inform you of the availability of orthodontic care and of the need to seek treatment by a qualified person. . . ." The individual advertiser may say the same thing but usually adds, "It's important to let *me* take care of your dental needs because I am open evenings, do better work, employ friendlier people, give out T-shirts with my name on them, etc."[17]

Diane Hughes, in her master's thesis, found that the success of practicing orthodontists depends more upon personality, propensity for risk, and need for recognition than upon rigidly applied business principles.[18]

Table 11

Use of Marketing Methods by Individual Practitioners (1985)

Method	Extent of Use
A. Seek referrals	
1. From dentists	
a. Letters of appreciation	80.4%
b. Entertainment	58.6
c. Gifts	52.3
d. Education of GPs	37.9
e. Reports to GPs	68.7
f. No-charge initial visit	50.3
2. From patients and parents	
a. Letters of appreciation	71.4
b. Entertainment	9.0
c. Gifts	17.0
d. Reduced-fee incentives	15.1
e. Follow-up calls after difficult appointments	57.3
3. From staff	43.9
4. From other professionals	30.5
B. Exposure	
1. Advertising—boldface listing	36.6
2. Active in community	53.5
3. Active in dental society	57.3
C. Supplying patient needs	
1. Office location	
a. Move office	27.2
b. Open satellite office	40.4
2. Office hours and scheduling	

a. Open some evenings	18.1
b. Open some Saturdays	17.8
c. On time for appointments	68.2
d. On-time finishing	54.7
3. More lenient payment arrangements	56.7
4. Cosmetic or comfort needs	
a. Lingual (invisible) braces	39.0
b. Clear braces	?
c. TMJ treatment	54.4
d. Functional appliances	63.8
5. Treat adult patients	89.2
D. Communication	
1. Office bulletin board	57.0
2. Practice newsletter	14.5
3. Patient education	43.7
4. Promotional gimmicks (T-shirts, jeans	?
patches, badges, diplomas, contests, etc.	

Source: "1985 JCO Orthodontic Practice Study," *J Clin Orthod* 19 (Nov. 1985): 805. Used with permission.

CHAPTER VI

Stabilization (1980s)

During the 1960s, certain politicians were concerned that, because of the rising cost of health care, a portion of the population was not receiving adequate care. They reasoned that, if the number of providers exceeded the demand, the cost of care would come down. Accordingly, the federal government increased its influence on the education of health care professionals, causing institutions to produce more practitioners.

In spite of these manipulations, by the 1980s health care costs were still rising, and more of the population were not availing themselves of health services. The idea had failed because a politically expedient solution was applied that did not take into account the demand for services.[1]

After these subsidies were discontinued, orthodontic class size began to come down. By 1980, the number of first-year students enrolled in orthodontic training programs was 283, having dropped from a high of 352 in 1972. For the next 12 years, enrollment did not vary more than 7% from the 283 figure, indicating that new-doctor output had stabilized. Furthermore, between 1982 and 1991, the ratio of orthodontists to general population increased minimally from 3.4 to 3.5 per 100,000. In California, the ratio actually fell (4.3 to 4.0).[2] These figures would seem to indicate that, at least as far as available patients were concerned, the outlook for orthodontists was at least not worsening.

Was the reduction in the number orthodontists being trained enough? In a variation on the theme played almost 10 years earlier by Robert L. Williams, Jack H. Okun, a Florida orthodontist, proposed that "if there were no new orthodontic graduates during the next 10 years, today's orthodontic specialty could easily handle the diminishing demand."[3]

FAVORABLE FACTORS

During any period of doom and gloom there are always a few who have words of encouragement. These words often have validity. One such individual was Robert R. McGonagle, president-elect of the AAO. In 1980, despite past surveys, he was optimistic. He reminded his constituents that "we have something nobody can take away from us, and that is our education." In addition, he listed 10 reasons for his optimism:

1. The increased use of preformed materials has helped compensate for the lack of substantial fee increases.

2. The efficient use of auxiliary personnel has enabled practitioners to see more patients per unit of time.
3. Incorporation and the adoption of Keough plans have helped protect orthodontists' earnings.
4. The output of graduate orthodontists has slowed.
5. There has been a 3 to 5% increase in the birthrate nationally.
6. A major public education program is underway that will tell the public about the needs and benefits of orthodontic care.
7. The AAO pamphlet, "3 to 7," distributed to pedodontists throughout the country, is being well received.
8. Adults—an untapped source of referrals—are now being encouraged to seek care through unsolicited newspaper and magazine advertising.
9. Many patients entering reception rooms would never have been there without third-party assistance.
10. There is evidence that administrators of such programs will recommend that their participants have the work done by board-certified or board-eligible orthodontists.[4]

Six years later, Arthur A. Dugoni added these words:

> Orthodontics is the fastest growing benefit requested by employees and implemented by employers, service corporations, and insurance companies . . . There will be approximately 52 million more adults, aged 18 to 74 years, with teeth who will be at dental risk in the year 2000 than there were in the year 1975. [Since adults were retaining their teeth longer, this foretold an increase in the adult-patient pool]. . . . In the 13 years between 1970 and 1983, the number of adults in specialty orthodontic practices increased from 5% to 24%.[5] The economic growth of dental care services between 1950 and 1982 exceeded the growth of the economy as a whole, medical care expenditures, and physician services.[6]

The implication was that, if dentists are busier, they are less likely to do orthodontics. Another favorable factor was the drop in first-year dental enrollment of 28% from 1978 to 1983.[7]

The AAO marketing program continued under full steam. The 1980s saw AAO representation on the radio series, "Consumers' Buying Guide," a monthly newspaper column ("Straight Talk on Teeth"),[8] TV and radio spots by former patient Dr Joyce Brothers, and a movie aimed at 10-to-16-year-olds ("A Special Kind of Dentist").[9]

At the state level, the Wisconsin Society of Orthodontists sponsored in 1989 a "Smile Day," whereby hundreds of "tin-grinned" youngsters were treated to an afternoon of professional baseball.[10]

ADVERSE FACTORS

In 1987 the AAO paused to evaluate its program thus far. Marketing studies revealed that:

1. Only 11% of consumers said they would consult an orthodontist first for advice on braces, as opposed to 78% consulting their dentist.
2. Two-thirds would prefer to hear about dental health issues and orthodontics from their general dentists.
3. Forty-one percent of general practitioners said that less than 15% of their patients needed orthodontics.
4. One third of GPs said they did some orthodontics, while 85% of pediatric dentists did so.

In other words, even though general public awareness had increased, potential patients were still not convinced that the place to start their quest for straight teeth was at the orthodontic office. What's more, there was still a communications gap between the specialist and the general dentist. Was the latter due to the AAO's current recommendation that only orthodontists treat orthodontic problems?

Terry McDonald, chairman of the AAO Council on Communications, certainly thought so. "We have to completely leave the who-should-treat issue," he said. "What we need to do instead is to promote the benefits of orthodontic treatment and what we can do as specialists to help our patients."[11] So the specialists' efforts to route potential patients around their general dentists had backfired; now they realized that they had bitten the hand that fed them. Under a new program, the AAO began distribution of a quarterly newsletter, "The Orthodontic Dialogue," designed to open the lines of communication with the GP and other referral sources.[12] The move came none too soon. "The antagonism between orthodontists and general practitioners who perform comprehensive orthodontic treatment is intense," observed Richard J. Smith, chairman of the Washington University Department of Orthodontics.[13]

In January 1990 the AAO held a special conference during which 120 association leaders examined 37 issues facing the specialty. Among the issues considered to be of a priority nature were: (1) specialty licensure, (2) OSHA, (3) availability of auxiliaries, (4) orthodontic education for nonorthodontists, (5) busyness/competition, (6) nonspecialist orthodontics, and (7) GP-orthodontist relations.[14]

While their leaders grappled with these issues at the administrative level, rank-and-file members were finding that patient care was but one facet of a specialty that was becoming more and more complex. As the decade closed, managed care continued to rise, corporations opened more clinics, and, as every niche of opportunity became saturated, orthodontists had to face the fact that there were only so many patients "out there."

CHAPTER VII

(1990s)

As organized American orthodontics approached its 100th year, it could look back on a century of achievement. From a crude, empirical "craft," the specialty had evolved into a technologically advanced discipline founded on scientific principles. It had embraced related sciences to increase its understanding and had broadened its scope from simple tooth moving to holism. It had become partners with other dental and medical specialties in order to give its patients the most definitive care. And its system of education had attracted applicants from around the world.

It had survived depressions, population shifts, intrusions of outsiders, and discord within its ranks (see Table III). It had also come to realize that certain things were not going to go away. It would have to live with managed care, government controls, nonspecialist orthodontics, clinics, oversupply, and opportunism for some time to come. John K. McGill and W. Charles Blair, DDS, who track the business of dentistry in their monthly *Advisory*, reported that "Orthodontics remains undoubtedly the most competitive segment of the dental profession. While the number of general practitioners offering orthodontic services had begun to decline, competition from pedodontists, low-cost clinics, and franchised operations had dramatically increased." They further pointed out that "most orthodontists have been forced to operate multiple facilities in order to maintain practice volume, resulting in the highest occupancy costs of any segment of the dental profession. . . . However, the biggest problem in orthodontics is the effect of the competition level on fee increases."[1]

Not at all convinced that "the number of general practitioners offering orthodontic services had begun to decline," J. Franklin Whipps, an Illinois practitioner, griped that, during his 20 years of practice, he had seen a "rapid growth of general practitioners doing orthodontics," and wonders how "the American Dental Association could, in good conscience, remain silent on this issue. The ADA certainly must realize that to fulfill one of its primary ethical guidelines, which is 'the competent and timely delivery of quality care . . . one needs more than limited training.'"[2]

Supporting that claim was T.M. Graber, editor of the *American Journal of Orthodontics and Dentofacial Orthopedics* and professor of orthodontics at the University of Illinois, who stated in a paper given at a 1996 AAO convention, that "one-third to one-half [of general dentists] are doing some orthodontics and the practice is increasing." Even orthodontic supply companies admitted that 55 to 65% of their products were sold to GPs and pediatric dentists, according to Graber.

Other "challenges to ethics" cited by Graber included "the problem of graduating orthodontists setting up with indebtedness of anywhere from $70,000 to $200,000, major financial commitments for equipment, and limited available locations. No wonder many take jobs working for Sears, 1-800-DENTIST, pedodontists, GPs, or Orthodontic Centers of America."[3]

For many in the audience, Graber's remarks hit close to home. Most of those present were "victims" of the clinic phenomenon and many were indeed participants. If you were a participant, you might get knowing looks from your peers, but at least you were doing orthodontics. As a victim, however, you might have seen a clinic opening down the street from your office and now it was doing "your" orthodontics.

Table III encapsulates some of the events having adverse effects (as envisioned by orthodontists) on their specialty.

Table III

A Chronology of Events Having Adverse Effects, Real or
Perceived, on Organized Orthodontics, to 1996

1929	Stock market crash, followed by Great Depression
1934	Orthodontics "at its lowest ebb"
1935	1st orthodontic advertiser in LA
1930s	Mail order orthodontic labs proliferate
1941	Outbreak of World War II
1945	1st LA orthodontic clinic
1945	1st organized "splinter" group (NYSSO)
1945	Fluoridation
ca. 1956	1st LA-area union-sponsored "clinic"
1957	End of postwar baby boom
1960	1st lawsuit over orthodontic society membership
1961	International Assn of Orthodontics incorporated
1964–75	Graduate glut
1965	*Unsafe at Any Speed* lends impetus to consumerism
1970	OSHA created
1972	1st official acknowledgment of busyness problem
1972	AB 1442 (Calif)—continuing education requirements
1972	Gov Reagan (Calif) announces capitation
1972	Title XI—loans for group practice
1973	Pres Nixon orders price freeze
1973	First dental PPOs
1974	AB 1455 (Calif)—extended duty functions
1975	Knox-Keene Act (Calif)
1976	FTC designates dentistry a trade
1976	1st department store dental center (Sears)
1977	*Bates vs Arizona*—advertising no longer unethical
1979–80	Inflation peaks at 16 1/2%
1980	Federal government encourages dental school enrollment
1982	AIDS diagnosed
1985	Gloves, etc., mandated
1987	OSHA Hazard Communication Standard
1987	Landmark lawsuit against an orthodontist
1989	HMOs move into dental market
1990	Major medical waste legislation
1991	Dr Acer accused of transmitting AIDS
1992	OSHA regulations
1996	Superclinics

One who might be called both a victim and participant was Sandra Kahn, who had a private practice in Pacifica, California. Kahn had to "work two other jobs just to cover costs." One of these was at a clinic where she saw as many new patients in a day as she did in her private practice in a month. What's more, Kahn did not agree with the notion that clinics do poor work. "I have learned to work fast and I know I can give these patients relatively good care even if I see 60 to 80 patients a day. . . . Let's face it, the attitude that clinics are not doing a good job is just denial on our part. Clinics have young orthodontists like me treating patients."[4]

SUPERCLINICS

A graduating orthodontic resident, Jeff Beyer, faced a similar dilemma, reporting in a June 1997 telephone interview, "The option of borrowing another $100,000 to start or buy a practice is certainly a scary proposition. The advent of [management service organizations (MSOs)] has provided a very tempting option for us [graduates]. At the AAO meeting, one company was guaranteeing $1 million net in the first 5 years of practice."

According to Gregory Oppenhulzen of Orthodontic Associates of Holland, Michigan, proponents of MSOs hoped that their concept would have the same effect on orthodontic care as the public had toward chain stores, in which McDonald-like organizations used "deep pockets and extensive media marketing to create name recognition and perceived value." They also envisioned a treatment database to ensure that patients would always be treated in the most efficient manner, like making an Egg McMuffin exactly the same every time."[5]

One such company was Dental Associates Limited, then operating six clinics in Wisconsin. They offered a guaranteed annual compensation of $135,000, with such benefits as liability insurance, health insurance, life insurance, investment plans, and continuing education.[6]

Another, and at that time the largest, "superclinic" was Orthodontic Treatment Centers Inc. OCA was founded in 1985 by Gasper Lazzara, a board-certified orthodontist, whose idea was to do for braces what Pearle Vision had done for eyeglasses. His $2770 fee was about 20% below the national average.[7]

The first publicly traded dental management company, OCA was operating, by September 1996, 180 offices in 25 states. OCA relied heavily on advertising directly to the consumer, using radio, TV, and newspaper advertising, and stressing convenience of location, expanded hours and days of service, toll-free phone numbers, and affordable fees. According to Blair and McGill, OCA spent about $56,400 per practice annually for marketing (*Forbes* says $72,000).

Typically, OCA provided capital for practice start-ups and acquisitions and provided all management services for affiliated practices, while the orthodontist had only to provide clinical services. Blair and McGill expected dental MSOs to reach a 20%–35% orthodontic market share within 5 years.[8]

Leaders in the specialty feared that many would answer the clinic challenge by becoming like them. "Do you want to spend $72,000 a year to see that your practice isn't going to the other guy down the street?" asks Graber, and calls this sort of thing part of the profession's "ethical and moral deterioration."[9]

PLUSES AND MINUSES

Other reasons for orthodontists' pessimism were:

1. "Back-door" orthodontists, Graber's term for those who work for pediatric or general dentists for a salary. The prevalence of this situation can be gleaned from the fact that, in 1995, over 40 general dental offices within a 20-mile radius of downtown Los Angeles offered specialist orthodontics.[10]
2. Patient complaints of impersonalization.
3. Staff turnover.
4. Persistence of motel courses for nonorthodontists.
5. Increasing popularity of courses dealing with the acquisition of patients; for example, a recent presentation, immediately preceding the PCSO Annual Session, was entitled "Uncovering the Secrets of the Power Practice."
6. Continuing government controls. The California Board of Dental Examiners had recently announced that, in order for dentists to renew their licenses, they must now complete, as part of their required 50 continuing education credits, four units in infection control and three in California dental law.
7. A recent AAO survey shows that 46% of respondents report that managed care was having a negative effect on their income and that 33% saw it as having a negative effect on their treatment decisions.[11]
8. Viewing the larger picture, public health professionals such as Dr Jay W. Friedman maintained that current managed care plans had not reduced the cost of care nor had they had any effect on the quality of care because of the lack of adequate surveillance mechanisms. They cited

the success of true HMOs such as the Kaiser Health Plan, which was based on large group practices of salaried GPs and specialists, comprehensive coverage, and good quality control.[12]

Not all observers agreed that the picture was pessimistic. What Del Stauffer, then ADA assistant executive director for health affairs, said in 1979 applied then: "What these clinics are doing is reminding people about dentistry who have never given the matter a thought before."[13] Eugene Gottlieb of the *JCO* said, "We are still living in the golden age of orthodontics," and cited these reasons for his optimism: "The orthodontist is still an entrepreneur, free to treat patients to his or her own standards, free to make all the practice decisions, free to make arrangements for treatment and fee."[14]

On the subject of MSOs, Gottlieb felt that "as long as a part of the public appreciates and will pay for the unique added value of a dedicated and well-managed private practice, the traditional orthodontic practice will survive."[15] Nevertheless, participation in managed-care programs continued to grow: Nearly 50% of orthodontists were so engaged, with PPOs having the greatest share.[16]

Despite the fact that the term *managed* care had become a dirty word in the dental vocabulary, orthodontists were forced to admit that the plans were coming up with patients who might never have materialized, while the clinics were providing jobs to recent graduates. And for the first time in history, compulsory office reviews were imposing standards from outside the profession.[17]

The latest AAO survey showed that, between 1986 and 1996, the average number of new-patient examinations per doctor had increased 23.8% and the number of new starts was up 41.4%.[17] This may have been due to what US Education Secretary Richard Riley called the "baby boom echo," referring to children of baby boomers. He said they represented the largest surge in school enrollment the country had ever seen and expected that the "echo" would be heard for at least 10 years.[18] H. Barry Waldman predicted a "major shortfall" by the year 2020 in the number of graduates needed to maintain the current orthodontist-to-population ratios. He cautioned, however, that this did not take into account the *demand* for services, the increasing number of adult patients, or treatment by nonspecialists.[19]

Blair and McGill were in agreement. According to their analysis, the number of doctors reaching retirement age would outpace the number of new graduates entering practice. They opined that the potential in orthodontic practice was "dramatic," due to more creative patient financing arrangements and increased direct-to-the-consumer marketing.[20]

On that score, the AAO marketing staff had not been idle. Their latest "coup" was the establishment of a national Orthodontic Health Month, as of October 1995. Included in the 1996 program were full-page magazine ads, national cable television advertising, and audio and video news releases to the broadcast media.[21] However, in May 1997 the AAO House of Delegates voted to phase out the yellow pages program. A study had shown that participants, after spending $1.2 million each year for the listings, got less than 2% of their referrals by this means.[22] For that matter, suggested AAO president David C. Hamilton, the current communications campaign had perhaps had limited success. As reasons, he cited "the lack of AAO's financial capability to adequately address or even marginally alter the public attitude" and "the too sophisticated and wordy message...."[23]

The state of orthodontics can be judged by many criteria. In this book, economics and freedom from stress have played major roles. What are we comparing it with? Orthodontics has fared better relative to other health professions with respect to managed care. On a worldwide basis, consider many European orthodontists, whose fees are set by the state. On the other hand, the present condition suffers by comparison with the golden age, but was the golden age the norm or a fluke? It may be that those who opened their offices during or just before the golden age simply fell into a good thing. Later, when normal market forces came into play, they began to get a taste of the real world.

Perhaps the "balance sheet" in Table IV will show that, like most occupations, the specialty can offer both good and bad. What is a better barometer than the intensity of competition for the 276 first-year places then (1995/96) available in graduate orthodontic programs?[24] Judging by the fact that there were 20 applicants for each place,[25] it seemed safe to say that orthodontics was still a good place to be.

Table IV

Orthodontics' "Balance Sheet" (1997)

<u>Assets</u>	<u>Liabilities</u>
Independence	Government regulation
Prestige, high income	Increasing overhead
Humanitarianism	Litigation
Challenging intellectually	Managed care
Outlet for manual skills	One-on-one relationship limits growth
Contribute to people's well-being	Frustration over unsatisfactory results
Develop pleasant relationships	Uncooperative or difficult patients/parents
Fellowship of congenial, educated colleagues	Competitive marketplace
Backing of strong organization	Isolation/"buck stops here"
Can delegate tedious tasks	Staff management problems
Career options: practice, teaching, research, public health, military	Limited mobility
Can work into twilight years	Exit barriers (disposing of practice)

CHAPTER VIII

Summation of PART ONE

Following a decade or more of plenty (known as the golden age of orthodontics), the specialty of orthodontics, beginning in the 1960s, was beset with certain forces that tended to affect the specialty adversely. The results of this study show that:

1. Some of the forces emanating from outside the specialty could have been offset, at least to some degree.
2. Those emanating from within orthodontics could have been offset to a greater degree, if not totally.
3. Some of the forces had both favorable and adverse effects.
4. The golden age may have been an artificially induced phenomenon based on fortuitous circumstances.
5. Although the effects of most of these forces persist, the specialty of orthodontics is still considered a desirable occupation and continues to attract aspirants.

Specific conclusions are:

1. *The declining birth rate.* To offset this, the number of new orthodontists entering the field could have been more carefully controlled.

2. *Mail-order orthodontics*, nonspecialist treatment, and motel courses. These long-standing grievances will not disappear. The problems can only be ameliorated by educating dental students about the complexities of orthodontic therapy and establishing better rapport with nonorthodontic colleagues.

3. *Managed care.* The insurance industry singled out dentistry because there existed at that time a combination of circumstances that made it vulnerable. These circumstances included
   a. A discrepancy between supply and demand
   b. Poor utilization of services
   c. Resistance of professionals to use marketing procedures
   d. Adverse economic conditions
   e. Adverse government climate[1]
Impact of managed care:
   a. Supplied additional patients to those doctors who signed up, but

b. Participating orthodontists had to accept lower fees.

c. In order to compete, many private practitioners resisted raising fees.

d. The prompt establishment of orthodontic service corporations might have been an effective barrier against the intrusion of managed care.

e. It is not realistic to expect an individual practitioner to ignore economic need, but prepaid plans could not have succeeded without employing "divide-and-conquer" tactics.

4. *Economic forces*
   a. Recessions. Not a controllable factor.

   b. Inflation. A dilemma. Had practitioners kept their fees in step with inflation, they might have been momentarily better off economically, but at the same time, they would have encouraged growth of the clinics.

   c. Consumerism. A movement that ultimately led to increased government regulation of professions (see Legislation).

   d. Office staffing. High turnover might have been minimized by taking a page from private industry and offering more pay and benefits.

5. *Government control.* Although nonpolitical factors such as clinics prevented orthodontic fees from keeping up with inflation, government efforts to lower fees did not succeed.

   a. Legislation. Because of complacency and noncohesiveness, the specialty failed to organize for concerted action, for example, to lobby against pending legislation.

   (1) Subsidies. Educators became overdependent on these and eventually found it nearly impossible to "turn off the spigot," resulting in doctor saturation, at least in urban centers.

   (2) Incorporation. Gave dentists financial incentives. Encouraged growth of clinics.

   (3) Extended functions. Permitted clinicians to delegate more duties, but led to depersonalization. Encouraged growth of clinics.

   (4) Continuing education. There is no evidence that CE legislation had improved competence or ethics.

   (5) Infection control. The use of universal precautions had reduced the possibility—but not necessarily the incidence—of infection, at least in orthodontic settings. Office overhead had increased, along with burdensome chores.

   (6) Aid to group practice. Newly formed groups hired some orthodontists, but most private-practice orthodontists were not busy enough to take advantage of government incentives. Encouraged growth of clinics.

   b. The Supreme Court

   (1) The ruling on advertising was beyond the control of organized dentistry and orthodontics.

(2) The AAO public relations and marketing program in response to the unbusyness of members was timely, ethical, and, for a time, effective.

(3) Even though the public has become more receptive to individual advertising, conservative members of the specialty were concerned that such practice tended to degrade the profession and lead to one-upmanship.

c. The Federal Trade Commission ruling on restraint of trade prevented two or more orthodontists from conspiring to boycott third parties. Nothing, of course, kept individuals from resisting.

6. *Litigation* might have been avoided to some extent by improved interpersonal relationships, use of informed consent, and better record keeping. This is corroborated by the proliferation of risk-management courses.

7. *Technology and extended functions.* The very developments that enabled orthodontists to treat more efficiently and economically, for example, bondable brackets, preadjusted appliances, and delegation of duties, are the ones that fostered the growth of nonspecialist orthodontics.

8. *Clinics*
a. Competition from clinics had driven down fees.

b. New methods of orthodontic care delivery, especially corporate, franchise, and publicly traded clinics, will continue to proliferate.

c. Depending on the doctor, it is possible for a patient to obtain good care in a clinic, but economic pressures militate against it.

9. *Nonspecialist orthodontics*
a. There is no evidence that patients receive better care from specialists than from nonspecialists.

b. The achievement of ABO status cannot be used as a criterion of competence when comparing specialists with nonspecialists because nonspecialists without university training (or its equivalent) are not eligible to take the ABO examination.

REFERENCES FOR PART ONE

(Please note: Parts One and Two are referenced separately and are formatted per the *AMA Manual of Style*, 10th edition.)

Chapter I: Early History of Organized Orthodontics

1. Casto FM. A historical sketch of orthodontia. *Dent Cosmos.* 1934;76:111-135.

2. Asbell MB. *Dentistry: An Historical Perspective.* Bryn Mawr, PA: Dorrance; 1988:176-177.

3. Weinberger BW. From "Irregularities of the teeth" to orthodontics as a specialty of dentistry. *Am J Orthod.* 1956;42:209-225.

4. Wahl N. Orthodontia's West Point: when Pasadena was the mecca for dental learning. *Southern Calif Quarterly.* 1992; 74(Summer):161-180.

5. Casto FM. A historical sketch of orthodontia. *Dent Cosmos.* 1934;76:125, 134.

6. Brodie AG. The Angle College of Orthodontia from the student's viewpoint, *A Memorial Meeting to the Late Edward Hartley Angle.* New York: Eastern Association of Graduates of the Angle School of Orthodontia, 1931: 22.

7. Lewis SJ. The development of orthodontic education. *J Am Dent Assoc.* 1934;21:1152-1165.

8. Fisher WC, ed. *Orthodontic Directory of the World.* 5th ed. New York: 1928.

9. Shankland WM. *The American Association of Orthodontists: The Biography of a Specialty Organization.* St Louis: The AAO; 1971:495-96, 757.

10. Asbell MB. A brief history of orthodontics. *Am J Orthod Dentofacial Orthop.* 1990;98:176-183.

11. [Omitted].

12. Casto FM. The trend of orthodontic treatment. *Int J Orthod Oral Surg Radiol.* 1930;16:1078-1092.

13. Asbell MB. Brief history. 208.

14. Oppenheim AJ. Tissue changes, particularly of the bone, incident to tooth movement. *Am Orthod.* 1911;3(October):56-67; 1912(January):113-132.

15. Asbell MB. Brief history. 208.

Chapter II: From the Depression to the Golden Age

1. Broadbent BH. A new x-ray technique and its application to orthodontics. *Angle Orthod.* 1931;1(January):45-66.

2. Brodie AG. Orthodontic history and what it teaches. *Angle Orthod.* 1934;4(January):85-97.

3. Weinberger BW. Historical résumé of the evolution and growth of orthodontia. *J Am Dent Assoc.* 1934;21:2001-2021.

4. Dewel BF. Orthodontics: midcentury recollections. *Eur J Orthod.* 1981;3:77-87.

5. Shia GJ. Business principles in an orthodontic practice. Part 1. *Am J Orthod Dentofacial Orthop.* 1986;90:253-261.

6. [Meeting of the] Southern Section. *PCSO Bull.* 1936(June):12.

7. *Los Angeles Classified Telephone Directory.* 1940.

8. Christen AG, Pronych PM. *Painless Parker: A Dental Renegade's Fight to Make Advertising Ethical.* Baltimore, Md: National Museum of Dentistry; 1995:297.

9. *Los Angeles Classified Telephone Directories.* 1935-1945.

10. Meinke H. A short history of dental advertising. *Bull Hist Dent.* 1983;31(April):36-42.

11. Soh G. The legalization of dental advertising in the United States. *Bul Hist Dent.* 1988;36(April):47.

12. *PCSO Bull.* 1938;14(September): n.p.

13. McCoy JD, McCoy JR. Organizing for pleasant and efficient practice. *Int J Orthod Oral Surg Rad.* 1930;16:29-41.

14. Waugh LM. Orthodontic appliances of laboratory origin. *N Y J Dent.* 1939;9(February):57-59.

15. Pollack HC Sr. Orthodontists and mail order diagnosis. *Int J Orthod Oral Surg Rad.* 1936;22:92.

16. [Meeting of the] Southern Section. *PCSO Bull.* 1934;10(September).

17. Shepard EE. Your organization: the American Association of Orthodontists. Paper presented at: 26th Annual Session of the Midwestern Society of Orthodontists; September 1963.

18. Harris NO. The struggle for fluoridation: a personal and historical perspective. *Bul Hist Dent* 35 (Oct. 1987):93-100.

19. Brodie AG. On the growth pattern of the human head from the third month to the eighth year of life. *Am J Anat.* 1941;68(March):209-262.

20. Downs WB. Variations in facial relationships: their significance in treatment and prognosis. *Am J Orthod.* 1948;34:812-840.

21. Björk A. *The Face in Profile: An Anthropological Investigation on Swedish Children and Conscripts.* Stockholm: Svensk Tandlaker Tidningen; 1947:40.

22. *Los Angeles Classified Telephone Directory.* 1945.

23. *Merriam-Webster's Collegiate Dictionary.* 10th ed. 1993.

24. Los Angeles Dental Society's own. *Bull Los Angeles Dent Soc.* 1969;13(May):7, 20.

25. New Jersey dental clinics to be regulated and licensed. *J Am Dent Assoc.* 1951;43:231.

26. Shankland WM. *The American Association of Orthodontists: The Biography of a Specialty Organization.* St Louis: The AAO; 1971:535.

27. McGonagle RR. Our golden age of orthodontics revisited. *Am J Orthod.* 1980;77:461–464.

28. Miner RM, Moorrees CFA. Retrospective. In: Ghafari JG, Moorrees CFA, eds. *Orthodontics at Crossroads.* Boston: Harvard Society for the Advancement of Orthodontics; 1991:239–247.

Chapter III: The Golden Age

1. Dewel BF. The journal celebrates its diamond anniversary: a remarkable record of achievement. *Am J Orthod Dentofacial Orthop.* 1990;98:1–4.

2. McCauley D. President's address, AAO. *Am J Orthod.* 1962;48:321–329.

3. Hillenbrand H, Dollar MM, Hudson AL. Prepaid orthodontic programs: a panel discussion. *Am J Orthod.* 1965;51:98–111.

4. Report of the AAO Qualifying Committee. May 1968.

5. Asbell MB. AAO. 71.

6. Salzmann JA. The threat of "social orthodontics" in prepayment programs. *Am J Orthod.* 1969;55:302–303.

7. H.C.P. (Pollock HC). It is here. *Int J Orthod Oral Surg.* 1936;22:305–306.

8. Brophy JE. Private and governmental programs for payment of orthodontic services. *Am J Orthod.* 1967;53:42–48.

9.Salzmann JA. Orthodontic planning in prepaid dental programs. *Am J Orthod.* 1966;52:56–58.

10. Orthodontics in prepaid dental programs (editorial). *Am J Orthod.* 1963;49:776–778.

11. Brophy JE. The American Association of Orthodontists and its role in prepayment programs. *Am J Orthod.* 1968;54:683–688.

12. Johnston WD. Orthodontic prepayment plans. *Am J Orthod.* 1969;55:286–293.

13. Hillenbrand H, et al. Prepaid orthodontic programs. 101.

14. Priewe DE. President's message. *PCSO Bull.* 1973;48(November):8.

15. FYI: Here's a quick look at managed care terms. *ADA News.* 1995(January):8.

16. Singer J. Managed care in dentistry. Lecture given at UCLA. June 9, 1997.

17. Schoen MH. External forces encouraging group practice. In: Green EJ, ed. *Dent Clin North Am.* Philadelphia: Saunders; 1972:265–274.

18. James AG. What is socialized practice? *J South Calif State Dent Assoc.* 1958;26(October):344.

19. Carter RD. Telephone interview by author, 10 Jul. 1995.

20. K.P.D. Discount dentistry and the new breed of advertisers. *Bull San Diego Co Dent Soc.* 1967(June):10.

21. Robbins MB. The case against closed panels. *Dent Manage.* 1968(July):32–45.

22. Prescott ML. The case for closed panels. *Dent Manage.* 1967;32(December):85–passim.

23. Robbins MB. 34.

24. Shia GJ. Business principles in an orthodontic practice. Part 1. *Am J Orthod Dentofacial Orthop.* 1986;90:256.

25. Graber TM. Auxiliary personnel: pillars of practice procedure. *Am J Orthod.* 1965;51:412–434.

26. Smith RJ. General practitioners and orthodontics. *Am J Orthod Dentofacial Orthop.* 1987;92:169–172.

27. We believe... *Int J Orthod.* 1962;1 (January):4–5.

28. Ricketts RM. *The Reappearing American.* Scottsdale, Ariz. Wright and Co; 1993:157.

29. McCauley, 327.

30. Evans T, Dittmann A-M. Orthodontic service: survey of need and demand. *J Acad Gen Dent.* 1974(November–December):25–28.

31. Brown WE, et al. How much orthodontics shall the pedodontist do? *J Dent Child.* 1958;25(1st qtr.):3–8.

32. Asbell MB. *The American Association of Orthodontists: A History, 1965–1990.* Unpub MS. 144.

33. Asbell. *American Association.* 146.

34. Brand IR. Dentist sues orthodontic group over membership. *Dent Survey.* 1966;42(July):21–22.

35. Pinsker vs Pacific Coast Society of Orthodontists and the American Association of Orthodontists. *PCSO Bull.* 1971;46(August):20.

36. Brand, 25.

37. Mage M. Early History of the American Society for the Study of Orthodontics. *J Am Soc Study Orthod.* 1966;3(May):33–34.

38. Jefferson Y. Remembering Leon J. Pinsker, DDS, MS. *J Gen Orthod.* 1995;6(December):5.

39. Pinsker LJ. Orthodontics... a sacred cow of dentistry. *Int J Orthod.* 1964;2(April):4.

40. Pinsker. Orthodontics... another key club? *Int J Orthod.* 1964;2(December):4.

41. Pinsker. The stainless steel curtain. *Int J Orthod.* 1964;2(January):3.

42. Shankland WM. *The American Association of Orthodontists: The Biography of a Specialty Organization.* St Louis: The AAO; 1971.

43. Shepard. President's address, American Association of Orthodontists. *Am J Orthod.* 1964;50:321–336.

44. International officers. *Int J Orthod.* 1962;1(January):2.

45. Challenge to the approval of the United States Dental Institute is pursued. *Orthod Bull.* 1974;3(November):3.

46. United States Dental Institute files suit against AAO and ADA. *Orthod Bull.* 1974;3(November):3.

47. $85.2 million suit filed against association. *PCSO Bull.* 1974;49(December):105.

48. United States Dental Institute litigation terminated. *Am J Orthod.* 1978;74:111.

49. Shia GJ. Business principles. 257.

50. Parker WS. Are our meetings functional? *PCSO Bull.* 1972;47(November):4.

Chapter IV: Decline

1. American Association of Orthodontists announces results of manpower survey, *Am J Orthod.* 1973;63:67–71.

2. Asbell MB. *The American Association of Orthodontists: A History, 1965–1990.* Unpub MS. 72.

3. Dewel, Population predictions, fertility rates, and professional prospects. *Am J Orthod.* 1977;72:93–95.

4. Gottlieb EL. Orthodontic economic indicators. *J Clin Orthod.* 1976;10:255–266.

5. Dewel BF. AAO constituent society presidents discuss current specialty issues: Part I. *Am J Orthod.* 1975;67:214–215.

6. Gottlieb EL. The growing economic crisis in orthodontic practice. *PCSO Bull.* 1977;50(September):30.

7. Court decisions alter the AAO: a report from the officers, trustees and legal counsel. *PCSO Bull.* 1979(Summer):24.

8. Asbell MB. *The American Association of Orthodontists: A History, 1965–1990.* Unpub MS. 12.

9. Shia GJ. Business principles in an orthodontic practice. Part 1. *Am J Orthod Dentofacial Orthop.* 1986;90:253–261.

10. Pinto D. The winds of change. *Dent Manage.* 1979(January);44:19–26.

11. *Los Angeles Yellow Pages.* 1975, 1980.

12. California Dental Association attacks use of earned degrees. *PCSO Bull.* 1973;48(February):47.

13. Shaping the future. *J Am Dent Assoc.* 1984;108:561–580.

14. *Federal Legislation Affecting Dentistry.* Hyattville, Md: Dept. of Health, Education, and Welfare; 1977:13.

15. Shaping the future. *J Am Dent Assoc.* 1984;108:561–580.

16. Simms RA. Prepaid orthodontic care today and tomorrow. *PCSO Bull.* 1975;50(August):11.

17. Brickner SL. Incorporation for physicians and dentists—1969. *PCSO Bull.* 1969;44(July):33–34.

18. *Federal Legislation.* 105.

19. Schoen. 270.

20. Watson WG. Challenges. *PCSO Bull.* 1974;49(August):5.

21. Gottlieb EL, Nelson AH, Vogels DS. 1985 JCO practice study. *J Clin Orthod.* 1985;19:863–870.

22. Questions about continuing education law. *PCSO Bull.* 1974;49(August):62.

23. Burakoff RP, Demby NA. Historical perspective and critical issues. In: *Symposium on Quality Assurance,* Vol. 29, No. 3, of Dent Clin North Am. Philadelphia: Saunders; 1985:427–436.

24. *Safety Pack.* Glendale, Calif: Safety Compliance Services. 1994), VI–1.

25. Pollack RD. Governmental regulations concerning infection control in dentistry. *Cur Opin Dent.* 1991;1(October):681–695.

26. Glenner RA. Sterility in dentistry. *Bull Hist Dent.* 1990;38(October):33–34.

27. Runnells RR. Countering the concerns: how to reinforce dental practice safety. *J Am Dent Assoc.* 1993;124:65–73.

28. *ADA Regulatory Compliance Manual.* Chicago: ADA; 1992:1.

29. Turpin DL. Infection control. *PCSO Bull.* 1987(Spring):4.

30. Drake DL. Optimizing orthodontic sterilization techniques. *J Clin Orthod.* 1997;31:491–498.

31. Bellavia DC. Efficient and effective infection control. *J Clin Orthod.* 1997;26:46-54.

32. Curley DK. Keeping up. *J Calif Dent Assoc.* 1990;18:12–17.

33. McLellan TS. Making a federal case: a perspective on government regulation. *J Mich Dent Assoc.* 1990;72(April/May):205–207.

34. Brophy. Private and governmental programs for payment of orthodontic services. *Am J Orthod.* 1967;53:42–48.

35. *The (AAO) Bull.* 1997;15(July-August):7.

36. The health care revolution: remaking medicine in California. *Los Angeles Times.* August 28, 1995:A16.

37. Asbell MB. *The American Association of Orthodontists: A History, 1965–1990.* Unpub MS. 115.

38. Dugoni A. Letter to the editor. *PCSO Bull.* 1983;55(Summer):12–13.

39. *What you should know about a managed care dental plan.* [Pamphlet.] St Louis: American Association of Orthodontists; 1996.

40. White LW. He that tooteth not his own horn. *J Clin Orthod.* 1997;31:81–82.

41. Letters to the editor. PCSO Bull. 1975;50(Feb):58.

42. AAO policy on relations between practitioner, patient, and carrier. *Am J Orthod.* 1974;66:211–212.

43. Friedman JW. The value of free choice in health care. *Med Care.* 1965; 3(April–June):121–127.

44. Poulton DR. Letter to Col W. E. Landfeld Jr. 15 May 1973.

45. Scholz RP. Letter to the editor. *PCSO Bull.* 1973;48(November):78.

46. Mermigas DC. Maxicare Health Plans Inc. In: Hast A, ed. *International Directory of Company Histories.* Vol. 3. Chicago: St James Press, 1992; 84–86.

47. Rudee DA. Letter to the editor. *PCSO Bull.* 1976;50(December):55.

48. Gottlieb EL. Hello! I'm your new partner. *J Clin Orthod.* 1997;31(April):205.

49. Dewel BF. AAO constituent society presidents discuss current specialty issues: Part I. *Am J Orthod.* 1975;67:214–215.

50. Members must not act to prevent PPOs from succeeding in the marketplace. *PCSO Bull.* 1984(Summer):33.

51. Antitrust laws, managed care, and you. *The (AAO) Bull.* 1997;15(January/February):2.

52. Sfikas PM. Unions in dentistry. *J Am Dent Assoc.* 1997;128:236–239.

53. Zernik J. Managed care—the Southern California perspective. *Am J Orthod Dentofacial Orthop.* 1995;107:19A.

54. Prescott ML. The case for closed panels. *Dent Manage.* 1967;85–86.

55. Cottingham LL. President's message. *PCSO Bull.* 1970;45(April):3.

56. Schulman ML. Orthodontic economic index. *J Clin Orthod.* 1981;15:466.

57. Position of the AAO on the delivery of dental care. *The (AAO) Bull.* 1984(March);2:2.

58. *Chronicle of America.* Mt. Kisco, NY: Chronicle Publishers; 1989:852, 867, 876.

59. Turpin. Orthodontic auxiliaries: in short supply. *PCSO Bull.* 1987;59(Winter):4.

60. A Survey of orthodontic auxiliaries. *PCSO Bull.* 1985;57(Winter):60.

61. Consumer protection. *New American Desk Encyclopedia.* 3rd ed. New York: Penguin Books; 1994:308.

62. Rubin RM. A crisis in orthodontics? *Am J Orthod Dentofacial Orthop.* 1987;91:508–509.

63. Burakoff RP, Demby NA. Historical perspective and critical issues. In: *Symposium on Quality Assurance.* Vol. 29, No. 3. Dent Clin North Am. Philadelphia: Saunders; 1985:427–436.

64. Asbell MB. *The American Association of Orthodontists: A History, 1965-1990.* Unpub MS. 163–164.

65. Recent litigation. *The (AAO) Bull.* 1988;6(January):3.

66. Sargeant RW. The defense of dental malpractice litigation. *PCSO Bull.* 1989;61(Summer):49.

67. Green CS. Good bites, bad bites, and malpractice suits. *J Am Dent Assoc.* 1978;96:13–14.

68. Holmes WR, Payne GS. Orthodontic malpractice claims prevention. *PCSO Bull.* 1985(Winter):38.

69. Rubin. 508.

70. Why every laboratory, every practice should offer orthodontics. *PCSO Bull.* 1976;51(March):48–49.

71. Christen AG, Pronych PM. *Painless Parker: A Dental Renegade's Fight to Make Advertising Ethical.* Baltimore: American Academy of the History of Dentistry; 1993:204.

72. Rosner JF, et al. Retail dentistry: practice and patient characteristics. *J Am Col Dent.* 1983;50(Summer):26–32.

73. Update on retail store dentistry, 1981. *J Am Dent Assoc.* 1982;104:498–500.

74. Pinto D. The winds of change. *Dent Manage.* 1979(January);44:19.

75. Glenn RE, et al. University of Iowa's study of retail dentistry raises some concerns. *Dent Econ.* 1982(February);32.

76. *California Department of Corporations Report* No. MISC1-061191. Revised July 22, 1991.

77. "Managing" managed care orthodontic plans using the quality assurance process. *PCSO Bull.* 1995;67(Fall):38–39.

78. *Dorland's Pocket Medical Dictionary.* Philadelphia: Saunders; 1989.

79. Moorrees CFA. Heritage paper. *Am J Orthod Dentof Orthop.* 1993;104:516–522.

80. Reid PR. Need versus demand for orthodontic service. *Am J Orthod.* 1967;53:414–422.

81. Dewel. Constituent society presidents discuss issues facing orthodontics: Part II. *Am J Orthod.* 1974;65:313–317.

82. Anderson GM. Years of change. *Am J Orthod.* 1964;50:521–527.

83. Moore AW. Orthodontic education: past, present, and future. *Am J Orthod.* 1976;69:42–56.

84. Kitchen WA. Message from the president. *PCSO Bull.* 1968;43(March–April):1.

85. *Acad Gen Dent News.* 1978(January):n.p.

86. Asbell MB. *The American Association of Orthodontists: A History, 1965–1990.* Unpub MS. 73.

87. Shia GJ. Business principles in an orthodontic practice. Part 1. *Am J Orthod Dentofacial Orthop.* 1986;90:253–261.

88. Dewel. Costituent society presidents discuss current orthodontic issues: Part II. *Am J Orthod.* 1978;73:340–344.

89. Garvin ME. Group practice. *J Can Dent Assoc.* 1953;19(July):91–92.

90. Grant P. History of the California health system. *California Hospitals.* 1990 (November/December, pt 2):51-52.

91. Salzmann. The threat of "social orthodontics'" in prepayment programs. *Am J Orthod.* 1969;55:302–303.

92. Dewel BF. Constituent society presidents discuss issues facing orthodontics: Part II. *Am J Orthod.* 1974;65:313–317.

93. Dewel. Constituent society presidents report on current orthodontic issues. *Am J Orthod.* 1976;69:340–344.

Chapter V: Reaction

1. Dewel. AAO constituent society presidents discuss current specialty issues. *Am J Orthod.* 1975;67:214–216.

2. Waldman HB. Changing number and distribution of orthodontists. *Am J Orthod Dentofacial Orthop.* 1994;105:128–134.

3. 1963–1984 Shaping the future. *J Am Dent Assoc.* 1984;108:561–580.

4. Dewel. Constituent society presidents discuss current orthodontic issues: Part II. *Am J Orthod.* 1978;73:340–344.

5. Shankland WM. *The American Association of Orthodontists: The Biography of a Specialty Organization.* St Louis: The AAO; 1971:503.

6. AAO Film huge success. *Orthod Bull.* 1974;3(July):5.

7. Asbell MB. *The American Association of Orthodontists: A History, 1965–1990.* Unpub MS: 84.

8. AAO National Communications Program approved in Washington, DC. *Orthod Bull.* 1979;7(July):1.

9. AAO embarks upon major public relations effort. *PCSO Bull.* 1979;51(Summer):23.

10. Asbell. *The AAO.* 90.

11. AAO public relations/advertising update. *Am J Orthod.* 1980;78:119.

12. Future of the AAO advertising program. *PCSO Bull.* 1983;55(Spring):32.

13. Yellow Pages—New look for AAO. *PCSO Bull.* 1983;55(Summer):4.

14. Shia GJ. Business principles in an orthodontic practice. Part 2. *Am J Orthod Dentofacial Orthop.* 1986;90:253–261.

15. Dewel. Constituent society presidents discuss issues facing orthodontics: Part II. *Am J Orthod.* 1974;65:313–317.

16. Lifschiz JM. Letter to the editor. *PCSO Bull.* 1985;57(Spring):9.

17. Turpin. Institutional vs individual advertising. *PCSO Bul.* 1981;53(Summer):4.

18. Hughes D. *An application of a classical model of competitive business strategy to the orthodontic industry* [MS thesis]. Philadelphia: Temple University; 1996:iii.

Chapter VI: Stabilization (1980s)

1. Daughtry CW. Marketing is a must for dentistry today, *PCSO Bull.* 1984;56(Summer):9.

2. Waldman HB. Changing number and distribution of orthodontists. *Am J Orthod Dentofacial Orthop.* 1994;105:129, 131.

3. Okun JH. Implications of the dentist/orthodontist ratio. *Am J Orthod.* 1987;91:169–170.

4. McGonagle RR. Our golden age of orthodontics revisited. *Am J Orthod.* 1980;77:463–464.

5. Dugoni AA. Future demands for dental care. *Am J Orthod.* 1986;89:520–521.

6. Dugoni AA. The economics of dentistry. *Am J Orthod Dentofacial Orthop.* 1986;90:78–80.

7. Okun. 169.

8. AAO Public relations/advertising update. *Am J Orthod.* 1980;78:119–120.

9. Richards R. AAO public relations activities. *PCSO Bull.* 1985;57(Winter):16.

10. Baseball, smiles a winning combination in Wisconsin. *The (AAO) Bull.* 1989(January):6.

11. AAO marketing to focus on referring dentists. *The (AAO) Bull.* 1988;6(July):4.

12. Asbell MB. *The American Association of Orthodontists: A History, 1965–1990.* Unpub MS. 95.

13. General practitioners and orthodontics. *Am J Orthod Dentofacial Orthop.* 1987;92:169.

14. Asbell. *The AAO.* 210–211.

Chapter VII: Present State of the Specialty

1. 1995 annual practice survey. *The Blair/McGill Advisory.* 1996(May):4.

2. Whipps JF. Letter to the editor. *Dent Econ.* 1996;86(July):16.

3. Graber TM. Professional ethics as we approach a new millennium. Paper presented at: AAO 96th Annual Meeting; Denver, Colo, 11 May 1996.

4. Kahn S. E-mail reply to "What's left for young orthodontists?" Retrieved from the Electronic Study Club for Orthodontics, University of Southern California, 9 Jun. 1997.

5. Oppenhulzen G. Management service organizations in orthodontics: a paradigm shift? *Am J Orthod Dentofacial Orthop.* 1997;112:345–349.

6. Letter from Dental Associates Ltd., Wauwatosa, Wisc. June 1997.

7. Dolan KA. Braces for the masses. *Forbes.* 1996;157(20 May):262.

8. Dentistry "goes public." *Blair/McGill.* 1996(October):3.

9. Graber. Professional Ethics.

10. *Los Angeles County Smart Yellow Pages.* 1995.

11. Survey results in on managed care. *The Bulletin.* 1996;14(July/August): 6.

12. Friedman JW et al. Rethinking dental insurance. *J Public Health Dent.* 1995;55(Summer):131–132.

13. Pinto D. The winds of change. *Dent Manage.* 1979(January);44:26.

14. Gottlieb EL. Rational expectations II. *J Clin Orthod.* 1996;30:183–202.

15. Gottlieb EL. Taking stock of management service. *J Clin Orthod.* 1997;31:407–429.

16. Number of orthodontists and orthodontic patients continues to increase. *The Bulletin.* 1997;15(July–August):7.

17. Singer J. Managed care in dentistry. Lecture given at UCLA, 9 Jun. 1997.

18. Magee M. Resounding "baby boom echo" means years of crowded schools. *Thousand Oaks [Calif] Star.* Sep.17, 1997:1.

19. Waldman. Personnel planning for the next generation of orthodontic patients. *Am J Orthod Dentofacial Orthop.* 1996;110:520–526.

20. Dentistry "goes public." *McGill Advisory.* 1996(May):8.

21. [AAO president] Hamilton DC. Mass mailing letter. 9 Sep. 1996.

22. Yellow Pages program to end. *Calif Orthod.* 1997(Summer):2.

23. AAO Presidents address house. *The Bulletin.* 1996;14(May/June):5.

24. American Dental Association Survey Center. *Surveys of Advanced Dental Education.* n.d.

25. Poulton DL. The future of the specialty of orthodontics. *J Calif Dent Assoc.* 1996(November):25–27.

Chapter VIII: Conclusions

1. Daughtry CW. Marketing is a must for dentistry today. *PCSO Bull.* 1984;56(Summer):8.

PART TWO

TWENTY-FIRST CENTURY

CHAPTER IX

Forces Outside Orthodontics

ORTHODONTICS ENTERS THE NEW CENTURY

As the millennial chronometer ticked off another thousand years, most of the world's inhabitants were hoping that the new millennium would bring peace, prosperity, and plenty. Instead, it brought a new woe: terrorism. The attack on the World Trade Center came to symbolize our new vulnerability. It was also a reminder that things were going on in the world beyond our cozy offices and that change was a given.

The biggest change was our job description. The practitioner had become more of a manager. We had become more defensive. Technology had become more firmly interwoven into day-to-day practice, both in managing the practice and in the performance of it. There were more gurus touting ways to deal with competition, economic decline, and increased litigation. The patient had taken greater control of his or her treatment. And there were more malpractice traps.

Despite these hindrances, the orthodontic boom that had begun around 1990 was continuing virtually unchecked. Since 1998, median gross income increased by nearly 19%. Between 1996 and 2000, the median number of case starts increased about 10%.[1]

According to Dr Leon Klempner, an orthodontic consultant, there were five major forces impacting private orthodontic practice by the second decade of the 21st century:

> ➢ Democratization of information: The Internet had both pluses and minuses.
> ➢ General dentists were no longer expected to be the primary source of new patients.
> ➢ Growth of midlevel providers: "super hygienists," competition.
> ➢ Newly graduated orthodontists had massive debt. They could not borrow money to start their own practices.
> ➢ Downward pressure on orthodontic fees due to the growth of dental service organizations.[2]

PATIENT SUPPLY

No indicator is more predictive of an orthodontist's prospects than patient supply. After a decrease in the ratio of orthodontists-to-children nationally from 1991 to 1995, it reversed course in '95–'96 to 17.7 orthodontists per 100,000 children in the same age range. To compensate, there was an increase in net income, allowing for inflation, from 1998 to 2005.[3]

In 2011, the birth rate was the lowest since 1920. The peak year was 1957 (double what it is now). A new low was recorded in 2016, when it reached less than 60 births per 1,000 women ages 15 to 44 (during the first quarter).[4]

Warnings such as, "Don't rest on your laurels," "Don't neglect potential adult patients," and "Inattention to the marketplace can be the downfall of an orthodontist," were given. One reason for the decline in the birthrate is that people of all ethnical backgrounds were gun-shy of marriage.[5]

GP ORTHODONTICS

In Their Purview?

Are general practitioners (GPs) really doing more orthodontics? R.N. Galbreath et al, writing in the May 2006 *American Journal of Orthodontics and Dentofacial Orthopedics (AJO-DO)*, didn't think so. According to their survey, most spent less than 10% of their practice time doing orthodontics (applies to comprehensive treatment) and this has not changed since previous surveys. Orthodontic treatment by pediatric dentists had declined since 1985, mostly treating crossbites, ectopic eruption, habits, postextraction supervision, and space maintenance.[6]

Gordon J. Christensen, prosthodontist and internationally known dental educator, believes that there are areas ordinarily defined as "orthodontics" that would not infringe on the orthodontist's bailiwick and advocates increased orthodontics by GPs. Some areas that fall within the realm of the general dentist's capability are

- Tipped teeth after adjacent extractions
- Collapsed occlusion related to secondary occlusal trauma
- Maladaption of a few anterior teeth
- Minimal malocclusions in the mixed dention[7]

Having Their Say

In a 2010 survey by Jim Du Molin, an Internet marketing expert for dentists, a number of interesting comments from dentists and orthodontists were received from both sides of the fence. They range from cautious, well-thought-out to nearly hysterical ("Would you send your wife to a family physician for her brain surgery?"). Three fourths of GPs think it's all right for generalists to do orthodontics, while only 4% of the orthodontists feel that way.

A sampling of comments from GPs who were in favor of GP ortho:

> ➢ "A conscientious general dentist who obtains readily available quality education in orthodontics is no less capable than any orthodontist in producing excellent orthodontic results."
> ➢ "I think GPs that do orthodontics are much more inclined to examine the occlusion during and after treatment than most orthodontists."
> ➢ "As long as they stay within their level of training and they refer when appropriate."
> ➢ "I've seen some fine orthodontics performed by GPs and many poorly done, misdiagnosed cases by orthodontists. It's the head and heart that drives the brackets, not so much the paper on the wall."

From GPs who were not in favor:

> ➢ "I have seen too many GPs influenced or trained by one guru. They do not have the arsenal of techniques that a good orthodontist has, thus providing the best of multiple solutions to an often complex situation."
> ➢ "General dentists don't have the proper knowledge to perform orthodontics. 'A little knowledge is a dangerous thing.'"
> ➢ "Most GP ortho CE courses are cursory and superficial. Only one or two are a true continuum that mimics an ortho residency."

From orthodontists:

> ➢ "... there is more to orthodontics than tooth alignment.... If these issues [function and facial esthetics] are not addressed, the alignment may be unstable, serious

functional problems can develop, and facial features can be compromised . . ."
> "With the advent of Invisalign, GPs are doing more ortho. Every orthodontist is being asked to help or bail out GP cases as they often underestimate the complexity of cases and/or tackling more complex cases than they should due to economic pressures. Very sad for our patients."
> "Orthodontics is deceptively simple to do. Any dentist can attach brackets and tie archwires . . . but knowing how to be efficient, accurate, and organized requires knowledge of biomechanics, growth and development, and other experiences one can only acquire with graduate study . . ."

And a pediatric dentist responded:

> "No different than a GP doing endodontics, prosthodontics, pedodontics, oral surgery, or perio."[8]

No Experience Needed!

To give you an idea of how dentists are being enticed into providing orthodontic treatment for their adult patients, the following paraphrases from a an article by Dr Rick DePaul are presented:

> Don't be afraid to provide orthodontic treatment for your adult patients.
> Anterior cosmetic correction in adults can be accomplished in 6 months by using the —— technique.
> Geared toward patients who don't want comprehensive treatment.
> Can minimize the amount of tooth reduction needed for veneers by opening the bite.
> Can minimize crown-lengthening.
> You can train at home.
> Average case fee: about $4,000 (as of 2015).
> Much of the work can be delegated to assistants.[9]

Do We Really Do It Better Than . . .

GPs? In a 2004 study comparing 126 models of patients treated by orthodontists with 70 treated by general practitioners, Abei et al found that a significantly lower (better) ABO Index score was achieved by the orthodontists.[10]

Pediatric dentists? Well, no. But not worse, either. A 2005 study by Mascarenhas et al compared the quality of orthodontic care between orthodontists and pediatric dentists when measured by the PAR occlusal index, treatment duration, and parental satisfaction. The quality of orthodontic care was found to be similar between orthodontists and pediatric dentists.[11]

Remember, however, these are just averages. Within your medical building, you might find unhappy campers on either side of the hall.

CORPORATE ORTHODONTICS—MSOs

Concept

Management service organizations (MSOs) are not new or unique to orthodontics (see Chapter XVII, Superclinics). Like any big business, MSOs are following the dollar sign. And the dollar sign is following markets that have high income potential. These corporations are aware that orthodontists are treating less than one fifth of the population that can benefit from orthodontic services. And they know that Americans tend to herd into national chain stores of every kind. The proponents of MSOs are hoping to have the same effect on the American mindset in regard to orthodontic care.

MSOs buy established orthodontic practices and, once purchased, the MSO owns all the tangible assets of the practice. Once the MSO owns a practice, it enters into a renewable employment agreement with the orthodontist, usually for approximately 5 years (6 months to 7 years). During that time, the orthodontist is generally paid a base salary plus incentives based on gross collections and overhead expenses. The orthodontist also signs a noncompetition covenant with the MSO should the orthodontist leave the practice.

One MSO wants to create a treatment database to determine exactly how to treat in the most efficient manner. It will use chairside computers, cost-based analysis, time-and-motion studies, and ongoing reevaluation to establish the precise, "cookbook" protocol to handle every aspect of the patient's experience. From the first phone contact to patting little Mary on the back as she leaves the clinic after debanding, the MSO will have protocols and frameworks that the practice must follow to perform optimally.

The MSO will have managers from the corporate headquarters who will be in close contact with the office administrators (office managers) in the practices throughout the country to oversee the practices. The advantage is consistency and efficiency, and it frees the orthodontist from some of the management headaches that many would prefer to do without. The MSO will provide health, life, workers compensation, disability, liability, and other forms of insurance. Staff incentive plans will be put into operation. Bulk purchasing and uniformity of supplies will reduce costs.[12]

Legality of MSOs

Dental MSOs are springing up to take advantage of this lucrative industry, and they range from simple entities to large corporate-owned operations, wherein a nondentist appears to be a quasi-owner. However, some states prohibit the ownership of dental practices by nondentists.

Running a corporate dental practice may provide certain tax benefits and shields from certain liabilities. However, some business models push the limits of legality. Therefore, both the decision to move into this model, and the actual transition, should be done under the supervision of professional counsel familiar with the unique laws involved.[13]

The late Peter M. Sfikas, chief counsel and associate executive director of the American Dental Association, reported a case involving a Chicago-area orthodontist, Dr Christine Michaels, as defendant in a breach of contract action brought by her MSO, Orthodontic Centers of Illinois (OCI), which was suing Dr Michaels for alleged nonperformance under her contract. OCI is a wholly owned subsidiary of Orthodontic Centers of America (OCA), a company that provides practice management services to orthodontic practices. An MSO typically takes one of two forms: either it will agree to provide comprehensive management services for a dental practice for a fee or it will purchase the practice from the dentist and them employ him or her either directly or indirectly.

Many states prohibit a nondentist from controlling or managing a dental practice. Other states expressly allow some level of ownership and control. The following two cases demonstrate the diverse approaches taken by district courts in different states and provide a background for the Michaels case:

In 2003, a federal district court in Texas, ruling against the MSO Orthalliance, held that it was a violation of the Texas Dental Practice Act for an MSO to own, maintain, or operate a dental office without a dental license issued by the Texas State Board of Examiners.

The following year, a district court in Georgia sided with Orthalliance in deciding the same issue under the Georgia Dental Practice Act. In this case, the court found that Orthalliance was not engaged in the illegal practice of dentistry, thus their agreements with the plaintiff orthodontists were valid.

Dr Michaels, like the plaintiffs in the Texas and Georgia case, sought to have her agreement declared null and void based on her contention that OCI was engaged in the illegal practice of dentistry under the Illinois practice act, convincing the court that OCI was engaged in the illegal practice of dentistry. The outcome of her case could compel courts in other jurisdictions to conclude that MSO contracts are unenforceable.[14]

One of the most unfortunate sets of circumstances in recent times involving failed MSO relationships concerns Dr Gasper Lazzara (also see PART ONE), an orthodontist-entrepreneur, and his companies Imagine Orthodontics, a nationwide chain of orthodontic practices, and its affiliate, Orthodontics Education Company (OEC). The lawsuits centered around the failure of Lazzara and his companies to honor contracts agreeing to pay graduating orthodontists tuitions and furnish jobs. OEC had agreed to put several students through school at three universities. In return, the students agreed that after completing their education, they would work for 7 years in an orthodontic practice owned by Imagine, receiving an annual salary of at least $150,000.

One of these students was Michael Sawaf. Sawaf completed his residency at Jacksonville (Fla.) University in July 2006 and moved his family to Brentwood, Tennessee, to begin practicing in a new facility owned by Imagine Orthodontics. He used a letter of employment from the company to take out a $500,000 mortgage on a home. But the practice never opened. Sawaf was asked to sign a note to pay $200,000 to reimburse his educational and living expenses, which he refused to do.

A few months later, Sawaf's attorney charged OEC/Imagine with violating its agreements, thereby absolving him of any financial responsibility. Thereupon OEC sued Sawaf and four other orthodontists for violating their educational and practice agreements, reportedly seeking more than $700,000 from each. Sawaf and another orthodontist then filed countersuits against OEC/Imagine and Lazzara.[15]

Another recent graduate, Ilan Abramowitz, was saddled with about $60,000 in education loans and a $500,000 house, but was not getting any salary nor could he work for another orthodontic practice without being found in breach of contract. He had a possibility of another job that would require a nearly 2-hour daily round trip. Ten students in the ortho residency program at the University of Colorado at Denver filed a similar lawsuit. Attorney Ronnie Bitman said that many of his clients were "stranded in cities where they have no friends, relatives or contacts. Many are without a paycheck and unable to feed their families or pay their mortgages or rents."[16]

Why Join an MSO?

To be a part of a new wave of orthodontic management that has been successful in many other businesses and so far is positioned to make each participant more successful; to prepare one's practice for a changing marketplace of clinic-based, high-volume dental centers; or to sell a large existing practice for a substantial, not otherwise obtainable, price.

Why *They* Joined

Jeffrey McMillan:
I was like many other new grads coming out of orthodontic residency. It's not uncommon for us to come out with tons of debt, some in excess of $500,000 to $600,000 or more in student loans. There's quite a bit of pressure to set up a practice right away, due to loan payments coming due. For me personally, I was apprehensive to borrow an additional $500,000 to $600,000 to face over a million dollars in debt load . . . then transition to my own practice.

Gerald Samson:
Being at the end of my career, and having been in private practice more than 30 years, what I was looking for was a way to transition my practice with the least amount of difficulty. What I had learned was to have a young orthodontist come in with me and build their practice within my practice, and then eventually I would transition out. After trying with two different associates, that just didn't work out for me . . . Joining a corporation turned out to be exceptionally attractive, because as part of the agreement, I could continue to practice in exactly the same way I had been practicing.

Adam White:
Most people start in corporate and then use that as a stepping stone to private practice, but what I did was the opposite. I moved from the private practice environment. Private practice hadn't worked out like I had planned for a number of different reasons, and having that dissolve a year and a half after my residency, I turned to the corporate orthodontic model.

McMillan:
Best suited for corporate orthodontics are newly graduated residents . . . also orthodontists in the twilight of their careers come to corporate orthodontics . . . they don't want the headache of running an office and dealing with all the things that are associated with the business end of a practice. On the other hand, orthodontists who have practiced a few years and have paid off their loans . . . may not be well suited.

White:

I think the person best suited for corporate orthodontic practice is one who is not particularly interested in having their name on the door. By the same token, the person who really wants his or her name on the door and has a deep interest in the business side of things probably would not do as well in corporate orthodontics.[17]

Comments from the Trenches

Generally positive

I'm looking for jobs and talking to Western [Dental Services, Inc.], and they ask me, "Would you have a problem seeing 80 to100 patients a day?" I say, "No problem." But the back of my mind says, "How the hell are you going to do that, newbie? Is the quality compromised? Do you get on [place a band or bracket] the sevens [second molars]? What mechanics are used to be so efficient? Do they just cherry-pick easy cases and send the hard cases away?"

I have worked at almost every office (when other orthodontists get sick, pregnant, etc.) Nobody else bonds sevens, the hygiene is terrible, and nobody seems to care, and they slop adhesive all over the teeth without cleaning it up. I would negotiate based on production—I am at 30%; most of the other orthodontists are higher at 33–35% . . . I went from school to 120 patients overnight at an OCA practice 7 yrs ago. It was horrible, but the pay was steady when I was first starting up. You can do it. You won't like it, but you can do it.

I've worked for Bright Now Dental for 10 years. I love it because the pay is good and I have full autonomy. I am the only orthodontist. I get to diagnose, treatment plan, and treat the patients from start to finish. I refuse to do phase I treatment on the majority of kids with mixed dentition and the company doesn't say anything . . . One complaint I have is they make me work an 8-hour shift (either 9–6 or10–7) when I can easily see all 60–80 patients in 5 or 6 hours; thus, there is a lot of free time between. In fact, I am working at Bright Now right now and still have time to type this post.

To save time and avoid emergencies, I don't do Herbsts or TADs [temporary anchorage devices]. I use Class II elastics. I extract upper 4s or 5s [first or second premolars], or upper 4s and lower 5s, depending on the severity of the Class II. I do band all the sevens, usually when I extract the fives or when I need to open up the deep bites. I think the treatment results at the dental chains are just as good as the ones in private practices.

Generally negative

Poor patient communication. Parents have a hard time calling the office after hours. Longer waiting time. Lack of instruments and supplies. They always run out of brackets, bands, and wires. All the cutters are very dull. I actually learn a lot from working under this nonideal condition. . . . learn to improvise and become more effective.

Expensive. Patients pay a lot for the mediocre customer service. They charge extra for broken brackets, for treatment extension, no shows, etc.

They pay you on collections, not production, at least here in the Southeast. At first, I had a $1,000 [a day] guarantee. This past year, it went to, I think, 28% of collections. So, I was figuring my paycheck went to about half. . . . We also ran out of stuff all the time. Basic mechanics only ... you have wires, brackets (sometimes), and elastics to work with. We did have power chain (yellow and purple). What? You don't want that color? Guess no power chain for you today.[18]

Impact of MSOs

Do they really cut into your business? Not according to Beverley J. Bunn's 2000 study in the AJO-DO. She found that within 2 years following the establishment of an MSO office, there was significant practice growth and improved business management and marketing by the traditional orthodontists in the vicinity. Most practitioners are reluctant to affiliate with an MSO, but corporate competition has actually increased case starts and comprehensive case fees. They have also educated conventional orthodontists about the importance of practice management and marketing.[19]

How can the private, noncorporate orthodontist best compete with the corporate model?

➢ Take advantage of buyers' clubs and consortiums to lower your equipment overhead.
➢ Your national, state, and local dental societies give advice on how to compete with Mr. Big.
➢ Independent orthodontists can do community outreach that many corporations aren't doing.
➢ The solo practitioner should not be trying to compete with a corporation. The level of customer service, knowing the individual patient, and offering more of a boutique service will make the solo practitioner successful.
➢ Offer a high level of orthodontics at a reasonable price. Keep in mind the single mother who is working two jobs

and wants her child to have straight teeth, but can't afford a big down payment and high monthly payments.
➢ Open a satellite office.[17] (See Chapter XIII, BUSINESS DECISIONS, Satellite offices)

Some caveats. Dr Jerry R. Clark, CEO of Orthodontic Management Group, advises: MSOs offer to provide management services for a fee. Although this can relieve the doctor of much of the business management, in most cases he or she gives up considerable control, and in many cases, is no longer the practice owner. When this happens, the doctor loses the critical element of why he or she became a private practitioner—the independence and freedom that comes from being one's own boss. Far more unpleasant to contemplate is what would happen if the management group were to be bought out by another company—or worse—goes bankrupt? Unfortunately, this has already happened to some of our colleagues.

Is the MSO a good exit strategy for an older orthodontist? Yes, but an uncertain one. In many cases, the doctor receives very little additional final reward for all the years of hard work spent building the practice.

Before you take such a drastic step, Clark recommends calling in a practice management consultant to help with financial, staff, or scheduling problems. Paul Zuelke, Hummingbird Associates, and Charlene White are good bets. Although when they depart, he cautions, the doctor and staff are often left to implement and carry out their recommendations. Other options: management teams, strategic planning, and environmental scanning.[20]

CHAPTER X

Government Control—Legislation

OCCUPATIONAL SAFETY AND HEALTH ACT

OSHA has been in place since it was enacted by Congress in 1970 to assure safe and healthful working conditions by setting and enforcing standards and by providing training, outreach, education, and assistance.

Infection Control

Orthodontic Products, in its March 2015 issue, offers a review of OSHA's infection control guidelines by means of questions and answers.

Q - Where are the greatest sources of infection in an orthodontic office?
A - Saliva splatters, splashes, and aerosols.

Q - What steps can be taken?
A - Infection control training for all clinical staff.

Q - Why does a practice need an infection control protocol?
A - Checklists, monitoring, and proper supervision ensure that all infection control and sterilization procedures are done correctly and are effective.

Q - What steps can staff take to minimize disease transmission risk during clinical activities?
A - Follow the Centers for Disease Control and Prevention (CDC) guidelines regarding
  - Immunizations
  - Hand hygiene
  - Purging water lines. Must be done daily for 2 minutes at the beginning of each work day and 20 seconds between patients
  - Proper use of barriers
  - Proper use of disinfectants. All containers of liquid must be labeled to prevent inappropriate use
  - Proper instrument sterilization. Sterilization bags must be dated after going through the sterilizer and has cooled off
  - Personal protective equipment

> ➤ Eyewash stations
> ➤ Aseptic technique

Q - What about common areas, such as the reception room?
A - Highlight the need for infection control in the nonclinical areas. Post a patient notice at the front desk such as, "If you have these symptoms (list flu symptoms) . . ." Put out alcohol hand sanitizers, tissues, and a trash receptacle, also pediatric masks for patients' siblings having respiratory infections. Other issues include unpackaged instruments, rescheduling "sick" patients, and appointing an infection control coordinator.[1,2]

Washington's Hazard-Prevention Program

The state of Washington's hazard-prevention program might be an example for other states to follow:

Dentists as employers must prepare a written policies and procedures (accident-prevention) program, and the initial hazard assessment evaluation must be reviewed annually. For all products used or stored, material safety data sheets (MSDSs) should be on hand.

Infectious waste management. Segregate infectious waste from regular waste. Personal protective equipment (PPE) must be worn at all times while handling infectious waste.

Standard precautions. In 1996, the CDC replaced universal precautions with standard precautions, which integrate and expand the concept, including hand washing, use of PPE, proper cleaning and disinfection of environmental work surfaces, and injury prevention.

Blood-borne pathogens, especially hepatitis B virus (HBV) and human immunodeficiency virus (HIV), should be high on the list of concerns for dental health care workers. Hepatitis C virus (HCV) is now included on the list, but no vaccine is yet available. In most states, gloves, masks, and eye protection are required when seeing patients at chairside (As of January 2017, the FDA no longer permitted the use of powdered gloves by health care providers when treating patients, because of health risks).

Hand hygiene is the single most important factor in preventing spread of pathogens. Wearing gloves does not preclude the need for hand washing. Washing of latex gloves is not recommended because it can result in micropunctures and subsequent wicking of liquids through undetected holes.

Sterilization and surface disinfection. Most instruments used in orthodontic practices are considered to be "semicritical," since they contact only mucous membranes but do not penetrate soft tissues. Because most items in this category— including handpieces and attachments—are heat tolerant, they should be heat sterilized between patients. If surfaces are contaminated, they must be cleaned and disinfected with an EPA-registered hospital tuberculocidal disinfectant. Keep in mind that disinfecting clinical surfaces involves two steps: cleaning and disinfecting.[3]

California's Program

New medical waste law. California's Medical Waste Management Act (MWMA) was amended in 2015. Its new regulations are broken down into three practice categories, depending upon whether a practice uses a mail-back system, it self-hauls, or one that only participates in a one-time event. Also included are storage times for medical waste. Further information can be found at cda.org/practicesupport.[4]

Hepatitis B vaccination. Within 10 working days of initial assignment to the job, Cal/OSHA requires an employer to offer the hepatitis B vaccination to employees who are occupationally exposed to blood-borne pathogens. The employer must also provide for postvaccination testing after the last shot. If that test is negative, another vaccination and testing must be offered.

PPE is considered appropriate only if it does not permit blood or other potentially infectious material to pass through employees' underlying garments or reach the skin, eyes, mouth, or other mucous membranes. If personnel wear scrubs as the uniform, then PPE must be worn over them. The employer must provide, repair, launder, and replace PPE.

Injury and illness prevention. Between October 2013 and September 2014, there were 29 citations awarded to California dentists for failure to have in place written plans for exposure control (blood-borne pathogens), injury and illness prevention, and hazard comuunication.[5]

Eyewashing. New OSHA regulations updated in 2015 state that "eyewashes must be capable of delivering tepid flushing fluid to the eye not less than 1.5 liters per minute for 15 minutes after a single movement and subsequent hands-free operation."[6]

Hazard communication. All employers must develop, institute, and maintain a written hazard communication program for the workplace. It must describe how the requirements for container labeling, safety data sheet (SDS), and employee information and training will be met. The written program must contain a list of the hazardous chemicals in each work area; who is responsible for the program; how the criteria for labels, SDSs, and training will be applied; and how the employer will inform employees of hazards of nonroutine tasks.[7]

Training. Dentists must take a 2-hour infection control course every license-renewal period (also see CONTINUING EDUCATION, below), provide blood-borne pathogens training to occupationally exposed employees upon hire, whenever a change in procedures might lead to increased exposure, but at least annually.[8]

Further information. The April 2017 issue of the *Journal of the California Dental Association* is dedicated to regulatory issues and has some excellent articles on infection control compliance and best x-ray practices. The journal can be accessed online by non-CDA members by going to the CDA Web site.

HIPAA AND OTHER PERSONAL INFORMATION

HIPAA Provisions

The Heath Insurance Portability and Accountability Act (HIPAA) Privacy Rule defines and limits the situations in which a covered entity (eg, an orthodontic practice) may use or disclose protected health information (PHI). State law may further limit the situations in which a practice may use or disclose PHI.

The Privacy Rule requires that a covered entity (that's you) provide PHI in specific instances to an individual or his or her personal representative when the individual requests (a) access to his or her information (release of records) or (b) an accounting of disclosures, and to the US Department of Health and Human Services when it is conducting an investigation, review, or enforcement action.

The Privacy Rule permits PHI to be used or disclosed without patient authorization for such topics as treatment, payment, and health care operations. Use or disclosure of PHI without patient authorization for public benefit and interest activities such as research, legal proceedings, domestic violence reporting, or disaster relief, may be done only under specific circumstances.[9]

HIPAA regulations are not violated if the patient has been informed how the doctor uses patient information and provides the collection agency only the minimum information for the agency to perform its task. In the contract, the agency must agree not to disclose further (say, to a credit bureau) patient information provided by the practice.

Broadly speaking, Social Security Numbers (SSNs) and driver's license numbers also fall under PHI. An orthodontic practice may collect these numbers for the purpose of confirming new patients' identity or their eligibility for government benefit programs, or because the practice is extending credit (agreeing to accept time payments). In such case, the practice must explain why the information is needed and how it will be kept safe. Businesses are prohibited from displaying SSNs on documents widely seen by others and from requiring patients to submit the information through unsecured electronic communications.[10]

Resources

A dental practice data breach can cost the dentist between $100,000 and more than $1 million. Those who have not taken the steps necessary to protect their patient data can take advantage of a kit published by the American Dental Association (ADA) titled *A Practical Guide to HIPAA Compliance* (members, $300; nonmembers, $450). CDA members can take advantage of the association's own "bundle" for $125, which helps practitioners design and implement a comprehensive program using a step-by-step approach.[11] For a more general guide not taking into account individual state laws, the American Association of Orthodontists (AAO) publishes a "Guide to Patient Privacy and Security Rules." (See also CHAPTER XII, Security, for additional discussion on data breach).

A Cybersecurity Checklist

These seven questions will help you evaluate your ability to protect your practice from security attacks:

> What would happen to your finances and reputation if private and personal information were stolen?
> Do your third-party vendors sign privacy agreements?
> Do you restrict your practice's social media account permissions and your employees' mobile access to work files?
> Does your practice have documented rules for cybersecurity?
> Do your employees report suspicious e-mails?
> Do you know your state's regulations for privacy breach notification?

> Do you have cyber liability insurance?[12]

AFFORDABLE CARE ACT

What's New?

There is nothing different or unexpected about how the ACA is rolling out as it relates to orthodontic care. The federal government has established "essential health benefits," which include medically necessary "orthodontia." It did not define "medically necessary orthodontia"; instead, it left determination to the states. The result is a patchwork definition because what may be considered "necessary" in one state may not be in the next.[13]

How Does the ACA Affect Orthodontists?

For patients expecting to be covered under medical insurance, inform them that benefits under dental insurance plans currently have not changed. Second, since medically necessary orthodontic coverage is limited to children under 19 and is one of 10 essential health benefits under the ACA, ask the parents to request of their medical plan "Which index does this plan use to determine medical necessity for orthodontic treatment?" In other words, encourage the patient to do the "tracking down." It is their plan. Most children, of course, will not qualify.

All measurements for the Salzmann and HLD indexes are done clinically—records are not necessary. Almost 85% will not meet qualifications. If your patient is among the other 15%, then take records and forward them for confirmation and review.[14]

TRUTH IN LENDING ACT

Your practice may be subject to the Truth in Lending Act (TILA) if you extend credit to patients or if you simply offer interest-free extended payment plans. Of particular note is the fact that if patients paying cash up front receive a discount for doing so, the amount or percentage of the discount is legally considered "interest" for those paying in installments and must be disclosed in the payment contract.

Orthodontists who regularly extend credit to their patients must comply with certain federal and state laws affecting consumer credit transactions. The most significant of these statutes for most orthodontists is the federal

TILA, which is implemented by the Federal Reserve Board through its Regulation Z.

Regulation Z applies to an orthodontic practice only if the following four conditions are met:

> Credit is offered or extended to patients.
> The offering or extension of credit is done regularly (ie, more than 25 times in the current or preceding calendar year).
> The credit is subject to a finance charge (ie, interest) or is payable by written agreement in more than four installments, and
> The credit is primarily for personal, family, or household purposes (ie, for personal or family orthodontic services).

Assuming that all the other conditions for coverage are met, a written contract for orthodontic services that is payable in more than four installments because of the installment pattern of paying, is subject to the TILA even if no finance charge is expressly added.[15]

ELECTRONIC HEALTH RECORDS

Dentists have been slow to adopt electronic health records (EHRs) in their practices but now that other health care providers have jumped on the bandwagon, dentists may be spurred to do so.

Benefits

Practice efficiency, patient communication and satisfaction, enabling practice expansion, and facilitating joining multidisciplinary teams.[16]

Legal Considerations

EHR solutions provide many potential benefits for dental practices, whether those programs run internally on a practice's computers or are cloud based. However, these programs also create new risks for a practice, which can be mitigated through due diligence and adequate contractual provisions to ensure protection for dentists.

The terms of a contract with a vendor providing EHR services entail a legal agreement with a vendor that is equally as important as the services themselves. Dentists must be assured that the storage and management of patient records is conducted in compliance with the HIPAA act of 1996 and its implementing regulations and other privacy laws.[17]

AAO members have access to legal and other resources online at https://www.aaoinfo.org. Nonmembers can obtain assistance, such as forms, from their state dental societies.

Typing 101

Our brethren in medicine "are deeply demoralized about the practice of medicine," according to Charles Krauthammer (himself an MD), writing in the *Washington Post*. They are overwhelmed by the "incessant interference" from insurers, lawyers, and government, turning doctors into typists, tapping data into a computer instead of caring for patients. One study found that emergency room physicians are spending 44% of their time filling out forms. If this is now happening to medicine, can dentistry and orthodontics be far behind?[18]

CONTINUING EDUCATION

Almost all states have continuing education (CE) requirements, ranging from 15 hours in Texas to 100 in South Dakota, per cycle, which varies from 1 to 5 years. The Dental Board of California's CE requirements, which are fairly typical, mandate that at each renewal period (2 years), the licensee must complete 50 units, not to exceed 25 units via online or home study.

Mandatory courses: Infection control, 2 units; California Dental Practice Act, 2 units; basic life support, 2 units.

Courses in the actual delivery of dental services: Courses limited to a maximum of 20% of a licensee's total required course unit credits (practice management, diagnosis, computers as pertains to dentistry).

Courses not eligible for CE credit: Money management, fitness, personal health, elective cosmetic surgery, and so forth.[19]

CHAPTER XI

Other Forces

PATIENT RELATIONS

One of the first things a newly minted practitioner learns is that there is more to orthodontics than straightening teeth. In addition to complying with government regulations, state dental board requirements, and dental society bylaws, he or she must see that the patient's total experience is a pleasant one—sore teeth being mostly unavoidable. The nice smile is a given.

Causes of Patient Dissatisfaction

Poor result, in the eyes of the patient—not yours.

Decalcification, white spot lesions, and caries. These can be avoided—or at least minimized—by insistence on strict oral hygiene and avoidance of cariogenic food and drinks. Bands must be checked at each appointment for looseness. Even intact bands may need recementation in cases of overlong treatment. Areas immediately surrounding brackets should be especially monitored in poor brushers.

Mechanical damage to teeth and supporting structures. Improper use of high-speed instruments, especially when used by dental assistants, can cause litigation-prompting enamel damage during adhesive removal.

Professional liability insurers must report all settlements and judgments to the National Practitioners Data Bank. That entity either provides a copy of the report to doctor's state dental board or instructs the insurer to do so. If the activity involved in the claim was disallowed by state regulations, an orthodontist is likely to face an investigation involving his or her license.

How to prevent:

> ➤ Doctors and staff should know the state dental assistants' regulations. Know what is allowed—and what is not.
> ➤ Doctors: Never assign a staff member to perform an activity that is disallowed.

> Doctors: Know what your staff is doing. Pay attention. Have frequent staff meetings to instruct and remind. Discuss the consequences of performing an unapproved activity, both to you and your staff.
> Staff members: Never perform an activity that is disallowed. Remind the doctor if such an assignment is inadvertently made.[1]

Root resorption. Probably the most common sequela resulting from orthodontic treatment that might be the basis for a complaint is external root resorption. It is not so much the occurrence itself, but how the orthodontist handles it that determines how the patient/parent will react. The best way to avoid a complaint—much less a law suit—is to:

> Take good records, especially radiographs.
> Make sure that your consent form includes mentioning the possibility of root resorption and that the patient or parent understands that resorption can occur even without treatment and that its severity depends a great deal on the amount of maxillary incisor retraction that occurs and the length of treatment.
> Take periodic X-rays of the maxillary incisors—more frequently if resorption was noted on the initial views or if treatment is prolonged. Keep patient informed of the root status. If resorption seems excessive, inform patient of the risks of further treatment and offer him or her the option of terminating treatment.[2]

Temporomandibular disorders (TMDs). The temporomandibular joint has always been the practitioner's no-man's land. One might say, Who's in charge here—the general dentist, the prosthodontist, the oral surgeon, the otolaryngologist, the psychiatrist, or the orthodontist? Theories about the cause of problems are as varied as the specialties involved. Is the cause anatomic, occlusal, neuromuscular, myofascial, psychological, or multifactorial?[3] Whoever is in charge, the orthodontist cannot be rightfully blamed for causing TMD because, according to a 1990 MEDLINE review by Reint Reynders, former research associate and clinical instructor at Northwestern University, sample studies indicate that orthodontic treatment is not responsible for creating temporomandibular joint disorders, regardless of the orthodontic technique, nor is orthodontic treatment specific or necessary to cure signs and symptoms of TMD.[4]

Social Media and Malpractice

Since the late '70s, when newsgroups, listservs, and chat rooms were competing for our attention, social media have changed the way we communicate—for better or for worse. With the appearance of Wikipedia, 2001 seems to be the kickoff year for social media. By 2004, we had Friendster, MySpace, and Facebook. Two years later, Twitter tweeted. As of 2015, the top two platforms were Facebook and Twitter, although MySpace was still holding on.[5]

Even if you yourself do not use social media, you can no longer ignore it. Comments, pictures, and personal information are continually being placed on a computer screen that may be accessed by people who will use the information negatively. It is difficult for any of us to know when we will need to make an impression and whom we will need to impress. If there are compromising images or information on a social media site, the impressions we make will be compromised.

When a patient consults with a plaintiff attorney about case viability, the attorney will peruse the professional's social media site for personal information about the doctor. Will he or she find personal pictures of the doctor in compromising activities or read information that is inappropriate for the role a professional maintains in the community? Every office should have a social media policy. Make it clear to the entire staff what may and what may not be posted on the practice's Facebook page, Twitter account, Linkedin, or other. Remember that HIPAA privacy regulations apply to social media just as they do to the office setting.

Elizabeth Franklin, claims manager of the AAO Insurance Company, warns that in litigation cases, attorneys can seize social media, so be careful what you put online. This can also apply to patients making false claims against the doctor.Orthodontists must be up to date on the trends and how to handle social media in their practices. A written policy outlines clear expectations, defines privacy policies, and assigns accountability when engaging in personal or professional social media on behalf of the practice. For example, only authorized individuals should be allowed to represent the practice on Facebook and other social media.[6]

Litigation

Why do patients sue orthodontists? The five primary elements of orthodontic treatment that contribute to making it highly susceptible to doctor-patient breakdowns:

> ➢ The protracted time period allows for problems and misunderstandings to develop and turn into dissatisfaction.

> Unrealistic expectations arising out of emotional issues are created and, if they are unmet, the disappointment and dissatisfaction may precipitate a lawsuit.

> If money is a problem for the family, or the family is attempting to "get something for nothing," sometimes the best defense is a good offense.

> Overlooked problems lead to lawsuits. One reason for orthodontic malpractice lawsuits is a problem with the treatment or outcome that was created by practice below the standard of care, for example, initial radiographs show shortened maxillary anterior roots, foreboding root resorption, but no progress images were taken.

> Inadequate communication. Communication issues may arise due to doctor's lack of listening or speaking skills, misunderstanding of patient expectations, critical treatment information not being conveyed to patient or parent, or lack of coordinating with other health care practitioners. In many cases, the parents are difficult to contact. They may be divorced, or they do not accompany the child to the office. In such cases, the doctor must leave phone messages, send e-mails, or letters and so document these, because the parents often deny hearing from the doctor.

The "deep-pocket" theory. Plaintiffs generally name as many defendants as possible to maximize the potential "pot" for a larger settlement or verdict. Resolving legal issues is arduous, costly, and unpleasant. Orthodontists should be mindful of developing problems with patients or parents and recognize their role in the process.[7]

Legal issues. Ten papers are available to AAO members from the AAO Legal Department (https://www.aaoinfo.org/legal-advocacy/legal-issues) to assist the orthodontist with 10 common issues: accidents, 20 legal questions, be careful what you promise, transitions, poor oral hygiene, informed consent, doctor-patient language barriers, adult orthodontics, overlooking pathology, and noncompliant patients with a bad outcome.[8]

The AAO Insurance Company receives at least one claim per month involving patients having tooth damage due to poor oral hygiene. One claim concerned a 16-year-old girl who was treated by two orthodontists at a clinic that had frequent staff turnover. After she was dismissed for poor cooperation and debanded, her general dentist noted that she was in need of 17 restorations. The family sued both orthodontists and the clinic, alleging that the doctors had failed to inform them of the poor hygiene and consequent caries. The second orthodontist did the right thing by terminating treatment, but by then it was too late.[9]

Donald E. Machen, orthodontist, legal consultant, and lecturer, sums up the reasons patients turn to litigation: failure to diagnose, failure to respond (which includes failure to treat, failure to refer, and failure to follow up); lack of adequate informed consent; poor, missing, or altered records; and treatment negligence.[10]

ECONOMIC CYCLES

As a result of the financial crisis of 2007–08 and the subprime mortgage crisis of 2007–09, the United States experienced the worst recession since World War II. The unemployment rate rose from 5% in 2008 precrisis to 10% by late 2009. Orthodontists were not exempt. During and shortly after this downturn, they could find no dearth of advice on how to cope with the economic downturn.

Rule Out Other Causes

Before blaming the recession, the practitioner facing a practice decline should also consider the following possibilities:

> Changing demographics of your area
> Case starts stay level or decline
> Not raising fees
> Your expenses go up
> Large number of patients paid up, but not finished
> GP ortho
> Drop in birth rate[11]

Some Coping Strategies

Dr Nelson. In the fall of 2009, *PCSO Bulletin* Editor Gerald Nelson offered these recommendations:

> Use that reserve account to bring you through the downturn
> Organize storage
> Revise scheduling protocols
> Assign marketing responsibilities
> Upgrade to a better computer system
> Install the X-ray machine[12]

Dr Sellke. Dr Terry Sellke, clinician, educator, and founder of *The Bottom Line*, tells us how to differentiate your practice, aside from faster and better: convenient hours and location, friendly service, run on time, and very convenient financing options. You must be actively involved in community activities. High staff turnover is a practice killer, he says, because "newbies" cannot deliver the care of a more experienced team member. It costs $30,00 every time you lose and replace an employee.

Other strategies: Find an underserved population, be a "niche player," create a "boutique practice," (eg, offer nail care and massages "while you wait"), offer Sunday hours, minimize your overhead, be an *acquisitioner* (buy out your competition).[13]

CONSUMERISM

The word has many meanings, but the one having the most devastating effect on orthodontics was the movement to protect and inform consumers by requiring such practices as honest packaging and advertising, product guarantees, and improved safety standards. Before the early 1940s, that definition didn't even exist, but by the mid-sixties, it had started gaining momentum. With the Truth in Lending Act, the government came into the picture. Now, with television and social media, it is a force to be reckoned with.

There has been a shift among the American population from being regarded as "patients" to one in which they view themselves as health care "consumers" with differing behaviors, expectations, and needs. This emerging consumerism is more salient in the younger population, who are more apt to prefer hi-tech interactions in which they can comparison shop through social media.[14] With a few simple keystrokes, shoppers can find the average cost of any dental service in their area through Web sites that compare the costs of specific procedures by ZIP code. They can accept the rate found on a Web site, negotiate for an even lower price, or pay cash and receive an even better discount. Patients are taking advantage of their improved bargaining position in part because of the increasing competition among private practices requiring differentiation through overall quality of experience rather than solely on clinical outcomes and new consumer-based services and products that can command a premium (eg, teeth whitening, digital restorative services, or orthodontic procedures for adults using aligners).[15]

What Hath Ralph Nader Wrought?

Has consumerism become opportunism? If you went to Google and searched for "Filing a complaint against an orthodontist," you would come up with 22,600 hits! It is easy to dismiss this challenge as a manifestation of those who are only too willing to take advantage of others' mistakes. But perhaps we have brought it upon ourselves by our failure to practice defensively, such as knowing that a disgruntled patient has plenty of advice on how to obtain satisfaction.

Advice to Patients, Step-by-step:

> Prepare your case: gather up your signed contract, e-mail messages, notes from appointments, for example; photos before, during, and after treatment.
> Speak with your orthodontist. Tell him or her why you are disappointed.
> Request that your treatment be resumed or continued at no charge.
> Request a peer review from the local dental society.
> File a complaint with the state dental board.
> As a last resort, explore litigation.

Cautions

> Keep copies of all communication.
> Be careful about posting negative messages on the Internet and other sites.
> Determine whether or not you wish to continue treatment with your current orthodontist.[16]

Advice to Doctors

If you receive a complaint from a patient or a regulatory body,

> Gather all pertinent information, including patient records.
> Contact your insurance claims representative.
> Follow instructions from your representative.
> DO NOT attempt to alter, add to, or delete any portion of patient's chart.[17]

STUDENT DEBT

How Bad Is It?

Between 2005 and 2013, student loan debt among all occupations nearly tripled, reaching an unheard-of $1.1 trillion for 37 million borrowers, and going back to '03, the percentage of 25-year-olds with such debt rose from 25% to 43%. By June 2013, it had reached such serious proportions that New York Federal Reserve Board economists warned that the burden of student debt could dampen consumer spending by that generation, as well as further hamper the recovery of the housing market and economy.[18] Five million Americans were in default of their loans. In fact, the overall student-loan debt is now higher than credit-card debt.[19]

An idea of what the aspiring dental or orthodontic student can expect in terms of costs can be gleaned from these statistics from the Orthodontic Alumni Association of Illinois newsletter in the winter of 2013. There were 72 accredited orthodontic programs in the United States that graduated 352 orthodontists annually. The University of Illinois at Chicago College of Dentistry tuition was around $65,000 per year for the orthodontic program. In 2010, debts of $250,000 to a high of $500,000 were reported from UIC orthodontic graduates.[20]

An August 2014 *Orthodontic Products* survey of orthodontic residents found that 22% expected to have less than $100,000 of student debt; 14% to have between $100,000 and $200,000; 24%, between $200,000 and $300,000; 18%, $300,000 to $400,000; and 22% expected to be over $400,000 in hock after graduating.[21]

What Can You Do?

If you see yourself as one of these unfortunates, here are some steps than can be taken (please keep in mind that these suggestions are taken from general publications and may not apply in every case)

> *Consolidate all your loans.* This will qualify you for forgiveness programs and make it easier to pay one monthly payment. It will also give you the opportunity to lower your monthly payment and extend the term of the loan. There are several possibilities:
>
> ➢ Check with your lender about a consolidation deal. Some lenders might want to keep your business for the long term.

> If you can qualify for private loan consolidation, here is a list of lenders:
> BND Student Loan Services
> Cedar Education Lending
> cuStudentLoans
> Next Student
> StudentLoan Consolidator
> WellsFargo

> The criteria vary, so ask the right questions:
> *Can I pay by debit or credit card without incurring a fee?*
> *Would I be paying a fixed or variable interest rate?*
> *Would I be subject to prepayment penalties?*
> *What is the discount if I make automatic payments from my checking account?*
> *What are the discounts for on-time payments?*

> Try one of the more than 130 credit unions in cuStudentLoans for a consolidation. Credit unions are nonprofit lenders, which means that you will probably enjoy the prospect of a lower rate and overall better deal.

> Consolidate your federal student loans into a Federal Direct Loan. Most recent loans should be this type of loan.

Apply for the income-based repayment program. The program will base the amount of your payment on your household income and number of dependents.

If you work as a teacher, you can qualify to have your student loan debt forgiven after 5 years. The TeachAmerica program or the AmeriCorps program also offer programs that can help you pay off your student loans.

Once you are employed, you need to set up a fairly tight budget that will limit your spending so that you have extra money to put toward your loan payments. Making the sacrifices now when you are used to being broke is easier than trying to cut back after you are used to spending a lot of money each month.[22]

What Can the Profession Do?

In a recent *JCO* report, Pruzansky, Ellis, and Park offered these suggestions to better prepare orthodontic students to face the realities of practice:

> Provide student-loan forgiveness programs.
> Control tuition increases.[23] (Some dental schools continue to increase tuition for orthodontic students while the same schools are paying oral surgery and other residents a livable stipend! [24])
> Include courses on financial planning in annual sessions.
> Offer more and stronger practice management seminars during residencies to review employment choices, contracts, and practice financing.[23]

INTERDENTAL RELATIONS

Ever since Edward Angle decided to specialize, orthodontists have been highly dependent on GP referrals. In a 2014 *JCO* survey of referring dentists, it was found that the most important factors in the GP-orthodontist relationship were the orthodontist's treatment results, patient satisfaction, and the orthodontist's reputation. Close behind was good communication about mutual patients, before, during, and after treatment. About three fourths reported that they would like the orthodontist to refer patients back to them for periodic checkups. They stressed a strong desire for written reports about their patients.

What Do They Really Think of Us?

Here are some typical comments:

> "Not enough orthodontists doing early orthopedic interceptive in my area."
> "Orthodontists must treat TMJ as well."
> "Why do some orthodontists not treat the second molars? I have braces off before the second molars fully erupt."
> "It would be nice to be kept informed of treatment so I could learn and better evaluate what is going on treatmentwise with the more advanced cases."
> "Send a note at the end of treatment."
> "Orthodontists should be acutely aware of occlusion and equilibration."
> "I never get any communications after the first treatment letter, and the letter is usually esoteric."

- ➢ "Orthodontists should be more aware of the perio status."
- ➢ "TMJ problems starting in their 20s. I refer to orthodontists who allow the maxilla to develop naturally and bring the mandible forward to match it, and who expand or distalize rather than extract."
- ➢ "Need more written records and photos. A phone conversation is a stress on my patient schedule and has too much detail to remember accurately."
- ➢ "They should be willing to treat minor tooth movements."
- ➢ "Free initial consults for patients are attractive."
- ➢ "Should stress need of periodic check-ups and prophies with the GP."
- ➢ "I see frequent root resorption and unadjusted occlusions."
- ➢ "Too many orthodontists have expanded too much the duties of their assistants."
- ➢ "I do not refer to an orthodontist if my patients have problems with excess cement or resin not cleaned off, wire problems, etc."[25]

CHAPTER XII

Forces Within Orthodontics—Technology

CLINICAL ADVANCES

Temporary Anchorage Devices

TADs are immediately loaded miniscrews and osseointegrated palatal implants placed to control tooth movement during orthodontic treatment and removed when the treatment is completed.[1] In "TAD, a misnomer?" Choo, Kim, and Huang point out that the description of TAD does not mention or describe anything about the skeletal component, which is the essence of contemporary mini-implant or miniplate systems. Perhaps a more appropriate catchphrase might be TSAD to reflect temporary skeletal anchorage devices.[2]

Eighty-four percent of orthodontists responding to a 2012 *Orthodontic Products* survey said they used TADS, and 8.1% added that they plan to start using them within the next year. The biggest obstacle to using TADS was a lack of training (74%): 35.4% of users delegate the placement of TADS to oral surgeons. Nearly twice as many orthodontists have received the training necessary to place them. The two most popular uses for TADS were molar protraction (58.0%) and distalization (50%). Orthodontists are using TADS, but they are using them sparingly; 72% use them for less than 10% of their cases.[3]

Distraction Osteogenesis (DO) is a surgical procedure used to reconstruct skeletal deformities and lengthen the long bones of the body. The bone is fractured into two segments, and the two ends of the bone are gradually moved apart during the distraction phase, allowing new bone to form in the gap.[4]

Used for several decades by orthopedic surgeons to repair long bone defects, DO has, over the past 15 years, gained acceptance for correction of various craniofacial deformities.[4,5]

Customized Orthodontic Treatment

Archwires. Perhaps a review of orthodontic wire history in Table V will put today's state of the art in perspective.

Table V

Orthodontic Wire Time Line[6]

1887	German silver introduced —actually copper (Cu), zinc (Zn), and nickel (Ni)	Edw H. Angle
Late 1800s	Arch bow—nickel-silver (Ag) or Platinum (Pt)-gold—.032" or .036" diameter. Had threaded ends	
1924	Stainless steel (SS) developed—"18 8" (18% chromium [Cr] and 8% Ni)	Wm H. Hatfield
1925	Edgewise appliance announced, having .022" × .028" slot for gold wires	Angle
1927	First to use SS	Lucien de Coster
Late '20s	Austenitic SS (Cr-Ni) alloy	
Early '30s	Annealed SS	
1934	Twin-wire appliance developed using two .010 SS wires	Jos E. Johnson
Early '40s	"Australian" wire developed, incorporating titanium	P. R. Begg (with A. J. Wilcock)
Late '40s	Elgiloy (Cobalt [Co]-Cr) developed for use in watches	Elgin Watch Co
1950	Orthodontic use for Elgiloy in 4 resiliences announced	Rocky Mountain Orthodontics
1960s	Gold generally abandoned in favor of SS	
1962	Nitinol (Ni-Ti, which exhibited "shape memory" at elevated temperatures) developed. Its name derives from **Ni**ckel **Ti**tanium **Na**val **O**rdnance **L**aboratory	US Navy
Late '60s	First to use Nitinol (50% Ni, 50% Ti) as orthodontic wire	Geo Andreasen
1970	"Straight wire" (along with bracket system)	Lawrence F. Andrews
Mid- 70s	Ti-molybdenum (β-titanium) had greater elastic range, ductility, and joining characteristics compared with SS, but had approximately 40% of its stiffness	
1980	TMA (titanium molybdenum alloy) "Superelastic" NiTi (Japanese NiTi and Chinese NiTi)	Chas J. Burstone & Jon Goldberg
1986		
Mid-90s	Cu NiTi	Rohit C.L. Sachdeva

Innovations began with light forces and heat-activated or thermal NiTi wires. Much has been done to nickel titanium (NiTi) archwires to vary the elastic forces within the same archwire. These wires are soft and pliable at room temperature, which permits easier insertion into the bracket slots. As the wire warms to mouth temperature, the wire becomes more "active." NiTi wire also has added resiliency and is available with curves of Spee and varying degrees of torque, as well as utility arch forms. There are also NiTi wires with surface coatings, which may reduce wire surface friction by 30%.

Beta Ti wire appears to be the intermediate wire between NiTi and stainless steel. This unique wire has half the force of stainless and twice the flexibility. In addition, beta Ti can be adjusted, within certain limits, to allow the clinician to individualize the archwire forms for each patient. Beta Ti permits asymmetrical arch formation and torque, vertical, and buccolingual bends, as well as rotation bends. Yet, even with these bends, it still has a certain degree of flexibility.

Another variation of copper NiTi, which permits insertion of a larger-sized archwire earlier in treatment is that it has a smooth surface, which is helpful in molar tube insertion. NiTi wires with temperature-sensitive, individual forces throughout the same wire have proven to be excellent for initial placement.

Customized systems—"robotodontics." In the past decade (apprx. 2002–2012), we have witnessed the development of new technologies in the fixed appliance arena, namely, Insignia (Ormco), orthoCAD (Cdent), iBraces (3M Unitek), and SureSmile (OraMetrix). These technologies enable clinicians to provide computer-driven, customized care at various levels. SureSmile, for one, is reported to have the potential of reducing the length of orthodontic treatment.[7] It is an all-digital system for orthodontic diagnosis, treatment planning, and fabrication of customized archwires, allowing clinicians to manipulate a 3-D, digital model of a patient's teeth and jaws to develop a virtual treatment plan by simulating orthodontic treatment. Wire-bending robots then fabricate orthodontic archwires with the necessary geometry to complete treatment according to the virtual treatment plan.[8]

Are they really better—or faster? A study by Saxe et al in the *World Journal of Orthodontics* used the standards of the American Board of Orthodontics (ABO) objective grading system (OGS) to determine the efficiency and effectiveness of SureSmile and found that it had a lower mean score (meaning that there were fewer points taken off), as well as a reduced treatment time compared with conventional treatment. The authors stated that the technique "has a great potential to both decrease treatment time and improve quality."[9]

In his master's thesis, Dennis J. Weber stated that Ormco's Insignia proved to be an effective tooth-moving application, based on the Peer Assessment Rating (PAR) score. Patients treated with Insignia turned in better ABO scores compared with patients similarly treated using conventional methods. Insignia was also more efficient in terms of treatment time and number of scheduled appointments.[10]

Is anybody using them? In a 2012 survey by *Orthodontic Products*, only 24.4% said that they currently use customized systems. The remaining 75.6% do not, reasons being cost and lack of proof of effectiveness. Of those who do, 49.2% reported using these systems in only 10% of cases they treat. Only 3.8% used them to treat 100% of their cases.[11]

Self-ligation

History. Self-ligating (SL) brackets are not new to orthodontics. In the mid 1930s, the Russell attachment was an attempt to enhance clinical efficiency by reducing ligation time. Some early SL brackets were the Ormco Edgelok (1972), Forestadent Mobil-Lock (1980), Orec SPEED (1980), and "A" Company Activa (1986). See Table VI, Orthodontic Brackets: A 101-Year Time Line.

Table VI

Orthodontic Brackets: a 101-Year Time Line

1903	Open tube appliance	Calvin S. Case
1911	Pin-and-tube appliance	Edw H. Angle
1917	Ribbon arch appliance	Edw H. Angle
1922	Modified Case's open tube appliance	Jas D. McCoy
1925	Edgewise appliance	Edw H. Angle
1929	Twin-wire appliance	Jos E. Johnson
1929	Universal appliance	Spencer R. Atkinson
1933	Begg appliance	Paul R. Begg
1935	Russell lock (1st self-ligating bracket)	
1950s	Bonded clear acrylic laminates, carved by hand	Geo V. Newman
Ca 1950	Twin ("Siamese") bracket	Brainerd F. Swain
1952	Suggested mandibular buccal angulated brackets	Reed A. Holdaway
1953	.018" slot	Cecil C. Steiner
1956	Lingual brackets (using	Glendon H. Terwilliger

	copper cement)	
1956	Tip & torque incorporated by soldering	Glendon H. Terwilliger
1957	Lewis bracket (rotation wings)	Paul D. Lewis
Ca 1960	Modification of Lewis bracket	Howard M. Lang
1959	1st torque bracket (anterior)	Ivan F. Lee
1960	Pretorqued and tipped bracket (anterior)	Jos R. Jarabak & Jas Fizzell
1963	1st commercial plastic bracket (GAC)	Morton Cohen & Elliott Silverman
1970	Straight-wire appliance	Lawrence F. Andrews
1970s	Clear, plastic (polycarbonate) brackets	Lee Pharmaceuticals
1970s	1st commercially available self-ligating bracket	Strite, Ltd
1972	Edgelok bracket (Ormco)	Alexander J. Wildman
1974	Lingual bracket (1st writeup)	Alexander J. Wildman
1975	Bimetric System	FF & GF Schudy
1976	Bioprogressive System	Rbt M. Ricketts
1976	First lingual bracket patented	Kinya Fujita
1976	Prototype lingual bracket	Craven H. Kurz
1977	SPEED bracket	G. Herbert Hanson
1979	Modified straight-wire appl.	Ronald Roth
1980	Ceramic bracket patented	James M. Reynolds
1983	Vari-Simplex System	Richard G. Alexander
1986	Tip-Edge System	Peter C. Kesling
1987	1st commercial aesthetic ceramic & sapphire bracket	
1990s	Reinforced polycarbonate (for plastic), polycrystalline alumina (for ceramic), and metallic slots introduced	
1996	Damon SL bracket	Ormco
1997	MBT bracket	RP McLaughlin, JC Bennett, and H Trevisi
1998	TwinLock	A-Co
2000	In-Ovation	GAC
2004	SmartClip	Unitek

SL brackets can be dichotomized into those with a spring clip that can press against the archwire (active) and those with a passive system of ligation, in which the clip, ideally, does not press against the wire.[12] *Do they save time?* Self-ligation appears to have a significant advantage regarding chair time, based on several cross-sectional studies as well as a small, but statistically significant, difference in mandibular incisor proclination. Shortened chair time and slightly less incisor proclinaton appear to the only significant advantages of self-ligation.[13]

Accelerated Tooth Movement

Both patients and practitioners want shorter treatment time and increased treatment predictability. Reduced treatment time limits possible risks and creates a more pleasant experience. Increasing predictability allows practitioners to treat more severe malocclusions in reasonable treatment times. Incorporating accelerated orthodontics (AO) into practice requires changing treatment planning and practice management systems. This is done by making changes in the alveolar bone through the biomechanics of applying force to teeth. AO modulates bone biology at the cellular level.[14]

Current therapies include local injections of biomodulators, laser therapy, mechanical vibration, gene therapy, and corticotomy, which act on or increase the expression of specific cytokines, chemokines, and growth factors (GFs). These molecules modulate the outcomes of orthodontic force application, accelerating orthodontic tooth movement (OTM), enhancing biological anchorage at specific sites, possibly decreasing the rebound effect, and assisting with the prevention of root resorption.[15]

Osteotomies and corticotomies have been combined with tooth movement to facilitate difficult tooth movements, reshape the alveolar arch, and accelerate tooth movement. Selective buccal and lingual decortication of alveolar bone has been used to accelerate orthodontic tooth movement (OTM). The theory behind accelerated tooth movement is that the corticotomy induces a response in the alveolar bone that can demineralize the bone around the dental roots. Once the bone has demineralized, there is a 3- to 4-month window of opportunity to move teeth rapidly through the demineralized bone matrix before the alveolar bone remineralizes. The bone response is called "regional acceleratory phenomenon" (RAP). It is similar to distraction osteogenesis, but less traumatic. Nevertheless, it is an invasive procedure, and whether it is worth it depends on how strong is the patient's desire for a shortened treatment period.[16]

In an e-mail to the author on December 27, 2016, Patrick K. Turley, UCLA professor emeritus, described another less invasive approach—in lieu of full thickness flaps with corticotomies—involving micro osteoperforations (MOPs), that is, making two or three small (2-3 mm) perforations in the cortical bone on either side of the teeth to be moved. This procedure is accomplished through the use of a popular device called Propel (Propel Orthodontics, Ossining, NY). The resulting area of inflammation recruits a cytokine cascade (ultimately, osteoclasts) that accelerate the rate of tooth movement.

Alikhani et al have stated that "micro-osteoperforations is an effective, comfortable, and safe procedure to accelerate tooth movement and significantly reduce the duration of orthodontic treatment.

Another approach involves wearing a mouthpiece that provides a light vibration to the teeth (AcceleDent). Manufactured by OrthoAccel, AcceleDent employs patented SoftPulse Technology that is said to speed up bone remodeling during orthodontic treatment by generating gentle micropulses to accelerate bone remodeling, thus enabling orthodontists to achieve more rapid and predictable clinical outcomes. The gentle vibrations have also been clinically shown to reduce patient discomfort.[17]

Decelerated Tooth Movement

Tooth movement can also be *slowed* by certain medications, such as hormone replacement therapy, nonsteroidal anti-inflammatory drugs (NSAIDs), long-term aspirin therapy, and osteoporosis medications, for example, bisphosphonates such as alendronate (Fosamax). Another good reason to take a thorough health history.[18]

Aligners

Ortho-Tain and its derivatives. In the early 1960s, Earl O. Bergersen, assistant professor of orthodontics at Northwestern University Dental School, in a nod to Kesling's tooth positioner, developed the Ortho-Tain as a finishing appliance. As opposed to the positioner, however, it was not rubber, but plastic; it was not black (or later, white), but clear; and it required no impressions or lab work. The principle was based on Bergersen's observation that there was a high correlation in patients' tooth sizes (large anteriors = large posteriors). Thus, the clinician, by measuring the widths of only the six maxillary anteriors with a special ruler and having sufficient appliances of different sizes on hand, could simply take one off the shelf and place it in the patient's mouth—not unlike fitting preformed bands from a box of 32 sizes. The Ortho-Tain was eventually available in 33 sizes.

A spin-off of the Ortho-Tain was the Occluso-Guide (1975), destined for the mixed dentition in 13 sizes, intended as a combination positioner, activator, and myofunctional appliance. A 2008 study in the *AJO-DO* found that "orthodontic intervention with the eruption guidance in the early mixed dentition is an effective treatment modality for occlusions with Class II or Class II tendency, excess overjet, deep bite, open bite, crowding, anterior crossbite, or buccal crossbite."[19]

In 1990, about the time the AAO started advocating age 7 as the ideal time for a child's first orthodontic exam, Bergersen came out with a preventive appliance (Nite-Guide) to be used in 5- to-7-year-olds to prevent crowding, overbite, and overjet from developing. (Letter from Dr Bergersen, January 19, 2004.)

Essix. The Essix appliance, invented by Dr John J. Sheridan and originally marketed by Raintree Essix, belongs to a class of thermoplastic retainers that also go under the names of vacuum-formed retainer and clear overlay retainer. Unlike the Ortho-Tain and Invisalign, it is fabricated for only one arch and snaps over the teeth. Although primarily a retainer, it is capable of minor tooth movements. Air-rotor stripping, another procedure pioneered by Sheridan, might be needed to gain interproximal space.

Invisalign. In 1998, Align Technology (Santa Clara, Calif) introduced Invisalign, a series of removable polyurethane aligners, as an esthetic alternative to fixed labial braces. The Invisalign system uses CAD/CAM stereolithographic technology to forecast treatment and fabricate many custom-made aligners from a single impression. Each aligner is programmed to move one or more teeth 0.25 to 0.33 mm every 14 days. This unique method of tooth movement has involved more adults with orthodontic therapy. In the past decade, Invisalign has been used to treat over 300,000 people worldwide, most of them older than 19.

As Invisalign continues to grow in consumer demand and professional use, questions regarding the efficacy of this system remain. How well do removable aligners move teeth? Align Technology reports that 20% to 30% of patients treated with Invisalign might require either midcourse correction or refinement impressions to help achieve pretreatment goals. However, many orthodontists report that 70% to 80% of their patients require midcourse correction, case refinement, or conversion to fixed appliances before the end of treatment.

Around the beginning of 2002, GPs could be certified in its use. Gordon Christensen encourages them to use it.[20]

Arguments and cautions against GPs using Invisalign:

> ➢ Patient satisfaction (they might expect more)
> ➢ High price for minor correction
> ➢ Multiple aligners needed
> ➢ Essix might be a better choice

- ➤ They basically tip teeth
- ➤ Many cases require auxiliary attachments (eg, bonds)
- ➤ Compliance issue[21]

While it may seem that the increasing availability of aligners would tempt more pediatric dentists and GPs to engage in orthodontics, there has been no proof—to this author's knowledge—that such is the case. What's more, the use of these appliances might create more awareness of both dentists and the public of the need for proper treatment as well as a new supply of patients whose treatment turned out to be unsatisfactory.

COMPUTERS

Applications

The introduction of computers into the field of health care has had an enormous impact on the way medical, dental, and orthodontic practices operate and provide patient care. From prediction tracings to bracket design, computers serve to simplify patient interactions, streamline record keeping, and improve diagnosis and treatment.

One of the major clinical applications of computers is in interdisciplinary orthodontics, wherein 3-D craniofacial imaging, digital models, and cone-beam computed tomography (CBCT) are changing our ways of imaging, diagnosing, documenting, and communicating between orthodontists and patients. Examples are multiple digitization or computer-aided point identification, image histograms to correct image problems, and smile analysis and smile design to aid orthodontic diagnosis and treatment. Esthetic smile design is a multifactorial decision-making process that allows the clinician to treat patients with an individualized, interdisciplinary approach.

The effectiveness of computer-assisted orthodontic treatment technology to achieve predicted tooth positions varies with tooth type and dimension of movement, so it behooves orthodontists to have a good knowledge of bioinformatics (collection, classification, storage, and analysis of biological information using computers).[22]

Digital Study Models

By 2013, digital study models were being used by 35% of orthodontic programs in US and Canadian dental schools. The most common advantage of plaster are the 3-D feel and the ability to mount them in an articulator. Advantages of digital models are ease of storage and retrieval and residents' exposure to a new technology.

The accuracy of digital model measurements was found to be valid, clinically acceptable, and more quickly obtainable.[23] The ABO now accepts pretreatment, interim, and posttreatment digital models provided in universal digital formats of specific orientation and internal construction according to specific guidelines. Posttreatment digital models are accepted only when accompanied by either plaster models or a 3-D printed stereolithic reproduction of the occlusal result. For further information, see ABO's "Digital Model and 3-D Printing Requirements."[24]

Digital models can be produced by either CBCT or an intraoral scanner. The former method is, of course, expensive and exposes the patient to radiation. The latter is more widely used and has the advantages of economy and compatibility with digital orthodontic systems and the ability to use these models to fabricate appliances.[25]

Security

Dentists must take the proper steps to make sure they aren't putting their patients and practices at risk in the form of crypto-ransomware, which attempts to extort money from dentists in exchange for their hacked patient records or the outright theft of computers and flash drives. In 2009, HIPAA was amended to extend patients' rights and the HIPAA Breach Notification Rule began. Since then, 1,400 incidents of a major data breach (an impermissible use or disclosure under the HIPAA Privacy Rule that compromises the security or privacy of patients' protected health information) have occurred.

In 2014, the California Attorney General's Office released its California Data Breach Report, which found that 70% of the health care sector that had breaches the previous 2 years were the result of lost or stolen hardware or portable media containing unencrypted data. In addition to criminal attacks that target the health care system, employees' use of unsecured portable devices is also increasing the risk of breach.

Recommendations

> ➤ Encrypt data at rest.
> ➤ If encrypting the data is not an option, strengthen the physical security of the server and hard drives.
> ➤ Password protection of computers alone is not secure.

HIPAA/HITECH regulations mandate that medical patient data being sent over a network be encrypted. That includes portable devices, such as laptop computers and flash drives.

> ➤ The entire office staff must use caution in accessing e-mail.

> ➤ Purchase a data compromise policy.[26,27]

Credit Card Terminals

"While cybercrime is well-documented, physical theft is still rampant, especially in dental practices, so it is important for dentists to protect their personal information as well as patient information," says The Dentists Insurance Company (TDIC) senior claims representative Rebecca Whitesel. Another threat lies in the fact that these smash-and-grab crimes expose dentists to future break-ins, as they give thieves firsthand knowledge of the practice's security measures—or lack thereof.

To prevent a break-in, TDIC recommends dentists consider the following precautions:

> ➤ Lock the terminal away in a secure location at the end of the day.
> ➤ Take the terminal home with you at the end of each day.
> ➤ Password protect your terminal, particularly for any refund functions.
> ➤ Upgrade your terminal to a self-disabling device, which requires the initial setup to be repeated if the terminal loses power. This also requires the issuing bank to be contacted in order to have your merchant number reassigned to the unit.
> ➤ Consider installing an alarm at your practice.[28]

DO-IT-YOURSELF ORTHODONTICS

Thanks to the Internet, particularly YouTube, orthodontists face a new threat—however small at present—do-it-yourself orthodontics (DIY).

Make Your Own Aligner

If you found out that a New Jersey college student used his university's 3-D printer to make his own aligner, you might raise your eyebrows.[29] But if you were told that homemade aligners were becoming big business, I suspect you'd raise your hackles. Two companies, SmileCareClub and CrystalBraces, now offer aligners for from $900 to $2100, depending on case difficulty. As of February 2015, SmileCareClub had signed up more than 90 orthodontists and dentists in 43 states to review photographs taken by patients and models made from homemade impressions. Oral health exam? That's also done by the patient, who signs a form to the effect that he or she has had a professional checkup with X-rays within the past 6 to 18 months.[30]

Gap Bands

Another popular DIY technique is the use of "gap bands"—rubber bands to close the anterior diastema (space between the upper central incisors). There is nothing new about this procedure, except its widespread popularity: A recent Google search of *gap bands* produced some 52,000,000 hits! You can now obtain orthodontic elastics from Amazon just as you could from Unitek or Ormco in bygone days.

Thankfully, many of these hits were warnings. One was from the editor-in-chief of the *AJO-DO*, Rolf G. Behrents, who cautioned that, because of the conical shape of these teeth, unsupervised use of this technique could result in the apical (rootward) migration of the rubber band, ultimately stripping away all the supportive tissue, and loss of the two teeth.[31] Have orthodontists helped to bring this plight upon themselves by advocating diastema closure? On the other hand, many celebrities, such as David Letterman, Madonna, Terry-Thomas, Condoleezza Rice, and Ernest Borgnine, have achieved fame despite their gaposis. It's a cultural thing, and most Americans have been brainwashed to cringe upon seeing it. But you watch and see. Some day that diastema—like tattoos—will become a badge of honor and Amazon will be selling separators.

A PERSPECTIVE

Every now and then, a sage comes along who helps us see our excesses. Perhaps we have been too enthusiastic about the powers of the computer and its technological magic. We are reminded that good craftsmanship is more than simply pushing buttons. Such a man is Robert G. Keim, editor of the *Journal of Clinical Orthodontics*, who said,

> When I look back at the accomplishments of orthodontists . . . who were trained prior to all the modern technological developments . . ., I notice that the results they achieved were not only equal to what we produce nowadays, but perhaps even better and more stable. I do not mean to imply that the myriad technological developments of the last 20 or so years are useless . . . but an overreliance on advanced radiographic techniques, superelastic archwires, and on-demand skeletal anchorage can result in a diminution of the skills and acumen of the individual clinician, who, in the final analysis, is responsible for the outcome of each treated case. It behooves

us all not only to stay abreast of scientific and technological developments . . . but to continually rededicate ourselves to honing our basic skills. Technology is no substitute for high personal standards and mastery of proven techniques . . .[32]

Chapter XIII

Practice Management

MARKETING

What They Didn't Teach You in School

It is no longer enough just to be good. To the public, that is a given. Like any other business, our practices are susceptible to changes in the marketplace. With the increasing number of dentists offering direct-to-consumer braces, aligners, and veneered "straight teeth," and the ubiquitous Internet offering a cornucopia of wares, prospective patients are now more keenly aware of their choices than ever before. It therefore behooves us to have a well-planned and well-executed marketing plan in place well before the consultation.[1]

Advertising

What's permitted. Effective May 2012 (and amended September 2104), AAO's marketing and communication materials may be used, that is, print, radio, TV, and banner ads; posters, educational fliers, and brochures; videos; and PowerPoint presentations. Materials must be unaltered except for the addition of doctor's name and photo, practice name, office addresses, office phones and fax numbers, e-mail and Web site address, practice logo, QR code, services offered, and appliance brands.[2]

Using a Web site. Today an orthodontic practice's brand is primarily defined by others. Social media provides a trusted, permission-based, highly scalable arena for sharing on a worldwide scale. Patients are talking about your practice whether you participate or not. Using a Web site as a dialogue platform with current, past, and potential patients allows a practice to be approachable and transparent.

Driving traffic to a Web site is very complex and depends on many factors, but three of these are within your control: (a) Your Web site needs to be up-to-date and accommodating to search engines. (b) Focus on publishing content. New search engine optimization requires participation on the part of the practice to publish genuine and original content—best through blog posts featured on the practice's Web site. (c) Possibly the most crucial step is harvesting reviews via Google or Yelp, accomplished by claiming, monitoring, and taking control of your Google+ page and having a consistent, effective means of getting reviews inside your practice.[3]

QR codes. QR codes were first used in Japan in 1994 and have been used internationally for several years. Standard bar codes have been around since 1974, but QR (quick response) codes contain much more data. In recent years, QR codes have got their impetus in this country from big brands such as Best Buy, Target, and Post Cereals. They are typically read by camera-enabled smartphones whose owners download a free reader application to scan the codes.

QR codes are easy to create (anybody can create them), and they are free to create. When you create a QR code, you determine where you want the code to send viewers—to a Web page, video, text message, coupon, or photo. How to use QR Codes in your practice:

> ➢ On traditional ads
> ➢ Posted outside your practice
> ➢ Posted inside your handout cards
> ➢ Inside your practice

QR codes are no panacea. They won't compensate for bad marketing. They are simply one more bullet in your online ammo belt.[4]

Consultants

During the Great Recession of 2007–09, orthodontists were the earliest and hardest hit group in dentistry; 75% of orthodontic practices had flattened or declined. The setback was serious enough to start many practitioners thinking: Orthodontics is not only a healing art—it's a business. Good businesspeople surround themselves with the right experts. They do four things better than doctors by:

> ➢ helping them achieve their goals more quickly
> ➢ having more experience than the doctors in their area of expertise
> ➢ being more objective
> ➢ keeping their client from making critical mistakes.

Patient and Doctor Referrals

These are the two most important types of referrals. To coordinate these patient sources, Dr Roger P. Levin, a leading dental consultant, recommends that the orthodontist hire a professional relations coordinator (PRC), who handles the administration, strategies, implementation, communication, and tracking of the referral marketing program. The time requires only 16–20 hours a week.[5]

Front Office Staff

Today, the Internet puts the consumer in control in a way that was never before possible. Jeff Behan, a marketing communications specialist, advised us in a 2008 issue of *Clinical Impressions*, that whenever consumers are interested in a product or service, they go to the Web as their primary source. Then, the first people that prospective patients see are your receptionist and front office staff. These individuals, perhaps more than any others, need to represent you well. If they can't represent the mission of your office in both personality and action, your practice will never convey that mission to the outside world.

Front office personnel need more than the ability to handle scheduling—and a smile that comes across on the phone. They must:

> Quickly determine whether prospects have been referred or are initiating contact on their own. Self-motivated consumers are not inclined to *give* a lot of information over the phone, but rather to *get* it so they can decide if you are worth coming to see.
> Make callers feel as though their call is the most important part of the receptionist's day.
> Uncover the basic reason that prompted the call.
> Handle questions about what makes you, your treatment approach, and your practice special.
> Clearly communicate the value of the consultation.
> Address any concerns the prospect may have.
> Gather information that may prove valuable to you and the treatment coordinator.[6]

Treatment Coordinator (TC)

> Confirmation call should be made by the TC and go to a cell phone.
> New patient appointment is 60 minutes and is entirely scripted.
> Procedure for a new patient tour of the office is also scripted, including the gift of a new electric tooth brush. Doctor is in the room for only 10 minutes. Then the TC closes the deal.

> TC results need to be measured daily. The treatment coordinator's start rate should be no less than 85% to 90%.[5]

How to Put the Internet to Work for You

Google search. Back in the early-to-mid-nineties, the first orthodontists to open a Web site to tout their practices got a leg up on their competitors. Now, having a Web site is as much of a necessity as is a business card. Ali Husayni, writing in the *Journal of Clinical Orthodontics*, tells you how to position your site so that it will come up before the viewer has scrolled through thousands of other sites.

Google uses an algorithm called a "spider" to crawl through all the Web pages and gives each a numerical rating, using more than 200 criteria. Husayni lists seven steps to make your site stand out:

> Put more information on your site.
> Rewrite texts copied from another site.
> Start a blog. The more you write, the more important you will look in Google's eyes.
> Optimize your site:
> Put key words, such as titles, headings, and copy in the right places.
> Remove any unnecessary background coding.
> Link one Web page to another.
> Strictly adhere to Google's webmaster guidelines.
> Register your practice in Google Places.
> Post positive reviews from satisfied patients.[7]

Social media. How to market yourself using a variety of social media sites:

> Add video to Facebook, such as office tours and new technology you are using.
> Share content about community events.
> Engage and interact with followers.
> Create ambassadors for the practice by treating every patient as though he or she were something special.[8]

Other ways:

> Make it easy to find your practice online.

➢ Encourage your patients to share their positive experiences online. Make sure the major review sites contain strong reviews.
➢ Find ways to differentiate your practice, for example, more doctor engagement.
➢ It's no longer good enough to produce an excellent clinical result—new and existing patients must see that your practice is special.[9]

Be aware of what's out there. Sometimes an article intended for consumers can be useful to a provider but it not only contains tips you can use to help sell your treatment, but it gives you an idea what you are up against. For example, an item titled "How to Save Money on Braces" is addressed to parents:

➢ Dental insurance— some plans cover a portion of the cost
➢ Start treatment early (may not always apply)
➢ Comparison shop
➢ Payment plans (eg, CareCredit)
➢ Pay total fee up front
➢ Treatment at a dental school
➢ Flex account money (from your employer)
➢ See if you qualify for free braces (Smile for a Lifetime Foundation, Smiles Change Lives program, etc.)[10]

Other Marketing Strategies

Internal. When the computer first became capable of printing Old English, I had a techie design an "Orthodontic Hall of Fame" diploma, which I awarded, from time to time, to a patient whom I felt was cooperative to an exemplary degree. It was fastened to a sturdy plaque, all ready to hang on the wall. Second only to the new smile, it gave the patient a long-lasting memento of a life experience (see Figure).

Roger Levin adds:
➢ Give away an Apple iPod or an iPhone every quarter.
➢ Treat one of your patients and 10 of his or her friends to a monthly pizza party.
➢ Throw out your new patient process and create a new one based on what your patients—not you—want.

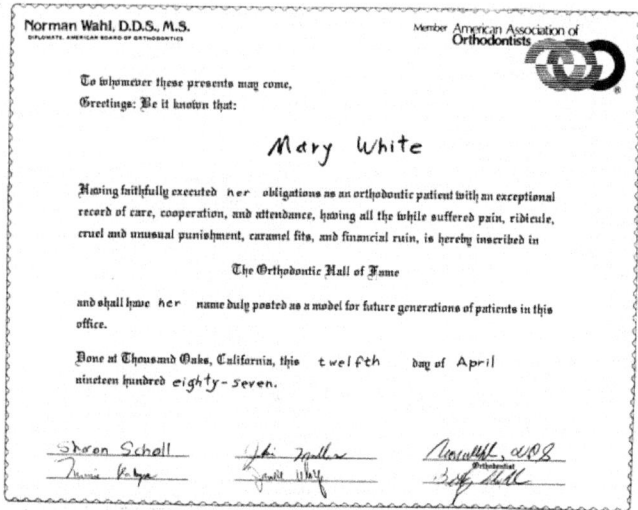

Norman Wahl, D.D.S., M.S.
DIPLOMATE, AMERICAN BOARD OF ORTHODONTICS

Member American Association of
Orthodontists

To whomever these presents may come,
Greetings: Be it known that:

Mary White

Having faithfully executed her obligations as an orthodontic patient with an exceptional
record of care, cooperation, and attendance, having all the while suffered pain, ridicule,
cruel and unusual punishment, caramel fits, and financial ruin, is hereby inscribed in

The Orthodontic Hall of Fame

and shall have her name duly posted as a model for future generations of patients in this
office.

Done at Thousand Oaks, California, this *twelfth* day of *April*
nineteen hundred *eighty-seven*.

Sharon Scholl

Figure. Sample diploma awarded to patient. Main inscription reads, "Having faithfully executed her obligations as an orthodontic patient with an exceptional record of care, cooperation, and attendance, having all the while suffered pain, ridicule, cruel and unusual punishment, caramel fits, and financial ruin, is hereby inscribed in . . ."

External (referring doctors). The percentage of doctor referrals in a healthy practice is 60% to 70%. Taking the occasional dentist to lunch will not induce them to send you patients. Quality relationships that involve multiple interactions will. Example: organizing an interdisciplinary treatment group. Getting good treatment results also helps. A study in the 2009 *Angle Orthodontist* found that 75% of responding dentists believed that occlusion and the functional result and patient satisfaction were equally important. Most respondents ranked canine guidance during mandibular excursions as most important, with Class I molar and canine relationships, even contact of all teeth in centric occlusion, and absence of balancing interferences also high on the list.[11]

What are your goals?

➢ Do you have a number for monthly production?
➢ Starts?
➢ The number of new patient exams should be designed to meet practice goals.
➢ No more than 2% of patients should be beyond their completion date.

> At least 98% of all patients should be booked for appointments.
> Is your overhead less than 49%?

Other pearls from Dr Levin:

> 80% of phone messages go to machines. Today (2010), 20% of people do not even have a land line. Your appointment reminders should go to cell phones and should also involve e-mail and text messaging.
> In a well-run practice, all patient interactions are scripted.
> Collect 99% of your billing. Patient financing is critical. CareCredit is strong in this area.

Call when payments are one day overdue.

> Measure your ratio of new patients to observation patients and your adult/child ratio.[5]

ORTHODONTICS AS A BUSINESS

Are Graduate Programs Doing Their Job?

In 2014, four fifths of orthodontic residents believed that their programs did an acceptable (36%), good (31%), or very good (14%) job of preparing them for the business aspects of owning a practice, but 19% of the respondents ranked their programs as poor (16%) or very poor (3%).[12]

Office Procedures

Consultation do's. Jeff Summers, writing in *Orthodontic Products*, offers these:

> Educate patients: Tell them how they can benefit from a new smile. After the consult, send the patient home with a professional packet of information.
> Respect people's time.
> Take advantage of Web-based consultation tools.

Consultation don'ts:

> Focus on selling. They're a captive audience, aren't they?
> Turn away young patients.
> Skip new patient records.

The key to a successful consultation is to establish a connection. Make prospects feel as though they can identify with you and trust you.[13]

Audiovisuals. Orthodontists need a public performance license to run a commercial movie in their offices. Under the concept of "public performance," failure to comply with the copyright law can result in penalties.[14]

Practitioners' missteps. Dr Ben Burris, writing in *The Progressive Orthodontist*, offers these missteps that practitioners most often make in connection with business management:

> ➢ human resources issues
> ➢ tax burden
> ➢ overstaffing
> ➢ overutilization of expensive technology
> ➢ investment mistakes
> ➢ failure to market effectively
> ➢ unwillingness to finance treatment
> ➢ inability to recognize change
> ➢ budgeting mistakes
> ➢ failure to save

Burris advises those who wish to add business acumen to their armamentarium to join study clubs that don't only talk about teeth, for example, the Continental Study Club, Schulman Study Club, and (Burris's) Progressive Orthodontist Study Group.[15]

Patient records. These include treatment notes, radiographs, models, photographs, billing records, and any other documents in the chart. Although these are the property of the practice, the patient—-and anyone designated by him or her—has the right to access the information contained therein, once a written request is presented. Whether it be the parents themselves or a third party, the authorization must meet both HIPAA and state requirements. AAO members can download an appropriate form for this purpose.

The practice may transmit copies of the record via unencrypted e-mail only if the patient consents after being informed of the risks of unsecure communications. A charge of 25 cents per page or 50 cents per microfilm page may be made, along with postage. Furthermore, the doctor may not deny access for reasons of unpaid bills.

In the case of divorced or separated parents, the noncustodial parent generally has the right to access a minor child's record regardless of whether the parent has custody or any financial responsibility. However, the orthodontist is not at liberty to release information to a parent without the minor patient's consent if it pertains to certain sensitive medical information such as pregnancy, drug abuse, or mental health. Nor need the practice release the records if the doctor has determined that such release will cause the patient harm.[16]

Practice aids. Management and marketing aids, such as a social media guide, Web content, forms, and releases, are available online to AAO members.

Associations

Many orthodontists do not have a written contract when they enter into an independent-contractor or employee agreement with another dentist or orthodontist. The orthodontist as a part- or full-time employee or independent contractor in a general dental or pediatric dental practice is becoming increasingly more common. Corporate dental service companies and MSOs are also aggressively recruiting dental professionals to work in their offices.

Beyond the handshake. In many such cases, the arrangement is launched with nothing more than a handshake. Unfortunately, without written documentation detailing exactly what was agreed to, if the relationship sours, there will be ambiguity, confusion, and higher legal fees. Consider this scenario:

> "Jane," a recent orthodontic graduate, facing $250,000 in student debt in addition to maxed-out credit cards, and unable to find a suitable orthodontic office needing an associate, is being interviewed by "Lester," a pediatric dentist in a nearby town. Lester says, "I'd be happy to have you work in my office as much as the demand warrants, and I'll pay you 45% of all receipts from orthodontic patients. You can also use my staff and equipment."

Jane quickly agrees, and on a handshake, begins making plans to begin her first job. Lester is too impressed by Jane's personality—and Jane is too excited by the opportunity—to insist on a written contract at this time. How could anything go wrong? Unfortunately, plenty.

Here are some questions left unanswered. The answers will not be found herein; they are best left to competent legal authority. Furthermore, each case must be judged individually.

> Is Jane an employee or an independent contractor?
> Will she be covered by the practice's liability insurance or must she purchase her own?
> In the case of nonpayment, missed appointments, or noncompliance, who has the final say with regard to treatment termination and other legal aspects?
> If the relationship breaks down, may Jane contact "her" patients to let them know of her new location?
> What was the understanding with respect to Jane's practicing nearby?
> May Jane take the patient records if and when she leaves the practice?[17]

In another example, a young orthodontist who had recently signed on with a corporate practice found out he was expected to place appliances on patients the same day they presented for consultation. In so doing, he would be unable to properly prepare a treatment plan based on a review of the records, discuss the plan with the patient or parents, or obtain informed consent. This was totally contrary to his training and what's more, he would be exposing himself to potential treatment problems, not to mention malpractice allegations. Unfortunately, divesting himself from the situation would be difficult, since he had just moved his family from another state.

Buyer Beware

A young doctor called her insurance company to report that she had just purchased a practice. After seeing several patients, she noticed a significant amount of root resorption and now wondered how to proceed. When asked whether she had "researched" the practice prior to purchase, she replied that the purchase opportunity had arisen quickly so there was limited time to do so. Now she was facing malpractice allegations early in her career.

The take-home message: Examine and evaluate as many of the patients you can, as well as their records:

Treatment records

> Do you agree with the patient's treatment plan? (There might not even be one!)
> Are there adequate records? Do they include a medical history?
> Has the patient been cooperative? How is the hygiene? Have incidents of these been documented?

> Is treatment progress commensurate with the estimated time?

Financial records. Chris Bentson, partner in a leading orthodontic valuation and transition service, suggests that you check these:

> the last 3 years' profit-and-loss statements
> the most current interim profit-and-loss statement
> the practice's tax returns for the past 3 years, including any other supporting statements
> the most recent tax year-end and month-end balance sheets
> a list of fixed assets
> production and patient starts for the last several years
> a list of active patients who are paid in full.[10]

Defending against allegations of practice below the standard of care—even though the care occurred before your "watch"—is expensive, painful, and time consuming. Don't let it happen to you.[19]

Satellite Offices

One of the ways orthodontists have sought to increase their patient base is to open a second office (and sometimes more than just one) at some distance away from their main office. This is by no means a recent strategem. Robert Strang, a 1906 graduate of the Angle School and the first orthodontist in Connecticut, opened a second office in Hartford because his Bridgeport office wasn't busy enough. He traveled by train 2 days a week. As the station was several blocks from his Hartford office, "sometimes it was run to the station or miss the train." (Could that be the reason he lived to be 101?)[20] In a study of satellite offices in the 2007 *Angle Orthodontist*, Heying et al came to the following conclusions:

> Orthodontists with multiple satellites start significantly more patients per year than do other practitioners.
> Satellite offices should be located ideally more than 10 miles from the main office.
> Multiple satellite practices tend to be more successful than practices with a single satellite.

Despite the ability of a satellite office to expand a patient base and increase net income, most practitioners would not encourage young orthodontists to establish a satellite office. One possible explanation is that the increased stress levels and complexity of operating multiple offices offset the expected profit increase.[21]

AUXILIARIES

Make sure your dental assistants are not doing procedures outside their bailiwick. If you practice in California, here's what she or he may do:

A Dental Assistant (DA) May
> ➤ take impressions for diagnostic and opposing models and sports guards
> ➤ place elastic separators
> ➤ remove separators
> ➤ take intraoral measurements for orthodontic procedures
> ➤ seat adjusted retainers and headgears, including giving instructions
> ➤ check for loose bands and brackets
> ➤ remove arch wires
> ➤ remove ligature ties
> ➤ light-cure bonded attachments

A Registered Dental Assistant (RDA) May
> ➤ remove excess cement from supragingival surfaces of teeth with a hand instrument or floss
> ➤ size [fit] stainless steel bands
> ➤ remove orthodontic bands
> ➤ place separators
> ➤ place and ligate arch wires
> ➤ take bite registrations for diagnostic models for case study
> ➤ remove excess cement from coronal surfaces of teeth with ultrasonic scaler (must have completed board-approved course)

A Registered Dental Assistant in Extended Functions (RDAEF) May
> ➤ take impressions for space maintainers, orthodontic appliances, and occlusal guards
> ➤ prepare enamel for bonding by etching
> ➤ remove excess cement from subgingival tooth surfaces with a hand instrument
> ➤ apply etchant for bonding[22]

Sick Leave

Orthodontists are advised to keep abreast of their state's current laws. In California, employers are required to grant their employees at least three paid sick days per year. Answers to such questions as the following can be obtained from your respective state dental board or dental societies (often, online):

> ➢ If I already provide my staff with sick time, must I pay an additional 3 days?
> ➢ I have been paying out unused sick time at the end of the year. May I continue to do so?
> ➢ Is this a required benefit for part-time employees as well?
> ➢ How can I keep my employee from abusing sick leave time?[23]

Leave of Absence

It differs from sick leave in that the employee is not paid, but is entitled to whatever benefits would otherwise have accrued, such as health insurance. Orthodontists should be familiar with the governing law, the Family and Medical Leave Act (FMLA), so that they can properly deal with an employee's request for leave of absence. There may be applicable state laws, as well. An example of a legitimate request would be an assistant's presenting a doctor's note indicating the need for an undefined period of time off for a medical condition. Other reasons might be care for a newborn or newly adopted child, care for a seriously ill family member, and employee's military service.

The leave of absence is used when the employee's time off from work is not covered under an employer's existing benefits such as sick leave, paid vacation, paid holidays, and paid time off. Upon receiving a request for leave of absence, the doctor should enter into an interactive process that involves a good-faith conversation with the employee to determine whether he or she can return to work following an injury or illness but can perform the essential functions of the job with reasonable accommodation.[24]

Overtime

Beginning December 1, 2016, employers must pay overtime to exempt employees who earn salaries less than $47,476 per year ($913 a week), according to the US Department of Labor new Fair Labor Standard's Act (FLSA) rules. Exempt employees are those who perform office or nonmanual work directly related to the management or general business operations of the employer.[25]

Meal and Rest Breaks

According to California's labor laws, an employee who works more than 5 hours per day must have at least one 10-minute rest break and a meal period of not less than 30 minutes. For a typical 8-hour day, she or he is entitled to two 10-minute rest breaks and a 30-minute meal break.[26]

Compliance

According to the California Department of Industrial Relations, successful compliance can be achieved by following these six steps:

> ➤ Display a poster on sick leave, leave of absence, overtime, and breaks.
> ➤ Provide written notice of these policies at the time of hire.
> ➤ Provide for accrual of 1 hour of sick leave for every 30 hours of work.
> ➤ Permit all eligible employees to use accrued paid sick leave upon request.
> ➤ Show how many hours of sick leave are available on the pay stub or document issued the same day as the paycheck.
> ➤ Keep records for 3 years.[27]

Employee Manual

The employee manual not only defines practice values, behavioral expectations, and workplace standards, but it provides employees with office policies, employee rights and obligations, safety regulations, and laws with which they are expected to comply. It guides the new employee through the difficult first days on the job, as well as serving as the "bible" of arbitration should misunderstandings arise between the staff person and the doctor.

The employee manual, or handbook, should include, among other things, the office policies on:

> ➤ requirements for appearance, including the dress code
> ➤ hours and schedule
> ➤ holidays, sick days, and vacation days
> ➤ salary, reviews, and raises

> ➢ use of PPE, when appropriate
> ➢ personal use of the computer
> ➢ use of the cell phone and other personal devices

Adherence to the policies should be understood by all employees and enforced equally by the employer. If a problem develops with a staff member, the orthodontist should be prepared to have an open discussion about her or his behavior. "By showing confidence and trust by involving the employee in the solution, not only will you likely get your desired result, you will have given the employee an opportunity to grow professionally and personally," says CDA practice analyst Michelle Corbo. Nevertheless, it should be emphasized in any written materials that employment remains at will and either party can terminate the relationship at any time.

Without an employee handbook, the practitioner is at a disadvantage should he or she face a lawsuit. Upon completion of the handbook, the orthodontist should have an employment attorney review it to ensure compliance with federal, state, and local laws.[28,29]

Performance Improvement Plan

Corbo recommends the following approach be taken in handling an offender:

> ➢ First nonserious violation: a gentle reminder of your practice policy
> ➢ Second offense: a sterner warning—a written reprimand
> ➢ Third offense: a final probationary warning that clearly asserts that any further offences are likely to result in dismissal.
> ➢ It is important to place copies of any instances of poor performance or disciplinary problems in the employee's personnel record. It is better to try to improve employee performance than to go through the painful process of termination.[30]

PRICING/FEES

The ideal fee—if there is such a thing—is one that makes the patient think he or she is getting a good deal and at the same time provides maximum profit for the practice. Dr Robert S. Haeger, a Kent, Washington, orthodontist, offers five pricing strategies from which practitioners can choose, depending on their practice style:

1. Market Pricing

Find out what other local practices are charging and set your own fees accordingly. Orthodontists are reminded that any agreement between two or more dentists with independent practices who agree on minimum or maximum fees or capitation amounts may be construed as price-fixing.

2. Two-phase Pricing

Haeger recommends determining the number of visits required to treat patients in two phases compared with full treatment. You can then calculate the revenue generated per visit. On average, two-phase patients need almost 9 more months of treatment and 10 more visits to finish.

3. Medical Pricing

In one form of medical pricing, set your fee high, even though no one actually pays that fee (it's called "Everybody gets a discount."). Then accept all insurance plans and pass the discounts on to the patients, offer a 10%–15% cash discount, and offer high discounts for sibling patients.

4. One Price Fits All

Set one price for adults and one for children. Insurance companies love such fee schedules, because the easy cases will subsidize the difficult ones. Of course, you might lose the simpler cases to competitors.

5. A Price Based on the Work Involved

This fee is more equitable for both patient and practice, because it creates a broad fee range based on case difficulty. The chief advantage is that you are not subsidizing the difficult cases with profits from the easy ones. Extra charges are made for missing laterals, missing lower second premolars without space closure, closing lower second premolar spaces with TADS, impacted canines, treating a 50% Class II, treating a Class II with a Herbst, and cases involving orthognathic surgery.[31]

EMERGENCIES

There is no better way to demonstrate concern for our patients than through our handling of emergency situations. Neal Kravitz, writing in *Orthodontic Products* in 2015, outlines his emergency protocol. Addressing patient concerns seriously, "I . . . make all effort to see the patient that same day . . . In today's consumer-driven society empowered by social media and doctor review sites where customer service reigns supreme, the orthodontist can no longer simply ask the patient to wait until their next appointment to be seen. . . . Never be too busy to pick up the phone."

> ➢ Respond immediately.

> ➤ Do not dismiss a patient's concerns.
> ➤ My time is not more important than my patients'.
> ➤ Do not charge the patient for broken brackets, no matter what.
> ➤ Schedule most emergencies before work, immediately after lunch, or even after work.
> ➤ If a bracket loosens on the same day as the bonding, always see the patient that same day.
> ➤ Keep a "hot list" ready to call emergency patients in case of a last-minute cancellation.
> ➤ Do not scold the child or lecture the parent. Assume full responsibility.[32]

PRACTICE SALE

Chris Bentson and Doug Copple of Bentson, Copple, and Clark have offered a step-by-step procedure for selling your practice, excerpts of which appear below. Even though you may have developed strong emotional ties to your practice after years of building and nurturing your "baby," it is nevertheless incumbent on you to approach this once-in-a-lifetime step with the cold attitude of a businessperson. Other than buying or selling your home, the sale of a practice may be the most important business decision you will ever make.

1. Gathering Knowledge and Strategic Planning
The most common questions that may arise are:
> ➤ Can you afford to retire? Many variables enter into an answer. A financial planner or your CPA can help.
> ➤ What will you do after you leave your practice? Will there be a void, or have you already starting thinking about that second "career"? Also keep in mind that people are living longer now.
> ➤ Where can you get help? Ask colleagues who have been through it. Get a list of practice transition specialists from articles in industry publications, the AAO, or the Web.

2. Practice Valuation
It will determine the current fair market value of your practice and will also serve to provide:

> ➤ a financial planning number you can incorporate into your retirement plan. You may find that you must work longer than you expected.

> a basis for making a transition plan, eg, how much will you pay the buyer when he or she becomes an associate and how much you are to receive when the shoe is on the other foot.

> an impartial figure of the practice's worth. It will be based on a valuation of at least the past 3 years of patient activity, financial data, real estate and other fixed assets, the demographic and competitive landscape, and practice history.

3. Finding a Buyer

For the past several years, it has been a seller's market. Data from the AAO's Practice Opportunities Online Service listed 452 doctors registered as practice seekers and 174 practices listing opportunities (including both sales and associateships). However, if your practice is not located in a relatively desirable area, such as a coastal town or large metropolitan area, it may take months or even years to locate a candidate.

4. Negotiations

The fourth step is to present to the potential buyer a terms sheet or letter of intent. This nonbinding document typically addresses the following points, among others:

> Who is selling and who is buying (the parties)
> Anticipated closing date
> What is being purchased (fixed assets, accounts receivable, etc.)
> Allocation of purchase price, as it has tax implications
> Payment terms
> Earnest money deposit
> Real estate considerations
> Noncompetition agreement
> Nonsolicitation of employees, patients, and referral sources

5. Legal Documents

The final step is to have an attorney translate the agreed-upon terms into a set of definitive documents to be signed by both parties.[33]

CHAPTER XIV

Risk Management

Over the past two decades, a new and complex pseudo-discipline has evolved: litigation and malpractice. The risk of litigation due to medical and dental malpractice is much higher in the United States than in any other part of the world. The orthodontist's need for legal protection has led to an increasing number of diagnostic procedures required to properly evaluate the pretreatment health status of the patient, thereby raising malpractice insurance premiums and the application of complicated, legalistic informed consent requirements.

Contributing to this confused situation are factors such as case reports describing severe sequelae that are nevertheless rare; contradicting studies; nonuniformity in approaching research questions; and, because of faulty reviewing processes, statistical or methodological flaws in studies that have found their way into publication. Because of this situation, contingency-fee plaintiffs' attorneys can manipulate the literature so that it will appear to substantiate their case to an uninformed jury.

The editors of *Risk Management in Orthodontics: Experts' Guide to Malpractice* state:

> Despite a lack of incontrovertible evidence of a direct connection between treatment and specific sequelae, studies have attempted to link orthodontically induced variables, such as treatment longevity, force magnitude, temporomandibular joint (TMJ) complaints, periodontal problems, allergic responses, and even post-treatment relapse, with the occurrence of various deleterious effects.[1]

PAYMENT DISPUTES

In the above book, Elizabeth Franklin, claims manager for the AAO Insurance Company, says that about half the litigation cases filed are settled, and the other half go to court. You have about a 50% chance of winning your case because the jury sympathizes with the unfortunate patient, not the wealthy doctor or the powerful insurance company. It is cheaper for the insurance company to settle the suit than to fight it, but your name is the one that appears in the National Practitioner Data Bank.

If you keep good records, follow the laws, and uphold the standard of care, your chances of being sued are greatly reduced. Like other doctors, orthodontists are depicted as affluent and likely to invite litigation. The public psychology is against us, so we must protect ourselves. Malpractice premiums have skyrocketed, spelling huge losses for insurance companies. In 2002, nine major companies stopped writing malpractice insurance because of their enormous costs.[2] However, there are steps to take both before and after you are likely to become grist for the malpractice mill.

> ➢ Screen the patient. Thoroughly evaluate each patient's ability to pay.
> ➢ Alternate payment methods. These could range from up-front payment of all or some of the fee to in-house financing to third-party financing.
> ➢ Address late-payment problems immediately. Waiting to allow the problem to correct itself rarely works. Make a friendly inquiry as to the reason. If the patient has not previously been delinquent, a second letter requesting payment may be in order.

Additional Measures

Despite phone calls and letters, an orthodontist can elect to continue treating the patient and not pursue any further collection efforts, continue treating the patient, but retain a collection agency or attorney to collect the balance, or terminate the doctor-patient relationship.

Do not:

> ➢ Meld the patient's treatment record with his or her financial or payment issues.
> ➢ Put the nonpaying patient on maintenance if that would not have normally occurred.
> ➢ Refuse to remove a patient's braces, if so requested, for nonpayment.

Dissatisfaction with Treatment

The patient may propose that the overdue balance be disregarded in exchange for the patient's agreement not to pursue a malpractice claim. In such a case, the doctor should seek advice from his or her professional liability carrier or personal attorney.

Collection Procedures

Should be part of your written office policy. They should include, at a minimum:

> - a time interval by which the account is considered delinquent
> - date when the first and second collection letters are sent
> - the form of these letters, when treatment is discontinued for nonpayment
> - how patients who are dissatisfied with treatment should be handled.[3]

Transfer Cases

Transferring out. With today's fluid population, every office should have a protocol for handling situations wherein a patient, because of a job change or other reason, must leave the area before treatment is completed. The first step is to make an appointment for transferring records. If the patient is in the early stages of treatment, these records should include, as a minimum, facial and intraoral photographs. Include radiographs if in the later stages of treatment.

Second, schedule an appointment with the patient or parents to discuss the financial aspects of the transfer. A common error is to simply multiply the completed fraction of the total time by the total fee and not factor in the cost of records, strap-up, and retention. A formula should be in place that is equitable for both parties. Dr Shawn L. Miller, writing in the June 2016 issue of *Orthodontic Products*, suggests that 25% to 35% of the total fee be allocated toward initial records and bonding, 45% to 55% toward treatment appointments, and 15% to 25% to appliance removal, final records, and retainers. Using these figures, the office can issue a check to cover future work. If, however, money is owed the doctor, under no circumstances should the records be held "hostage" in an effort to collect.

Finally, the new orthodontist should be provided with the treatment particulars, after HIPAA release. The AAO has an editable standard form that can be downloaded from their Web site that includes diagnosis, treatment plan, appliances and mechanics used, and other pertinent facts. A final consultation should be scheduled during which the case progress should be reviewed and an opportunity given for patient questions. The probability that the new doctor's treatment approach will differ from yours should be mentioned. By all means, any unusual circumstances, such as failure to meet progress goals, should be noted so that no surprises will surface at the other end. For your legal protection, such statements should be carefully documented. This appointment can also be the opportunity to create goodwill.

Transferring in. Accepting a transfer patient can be not only a source of future referrals, but it casts a favorable light on the specialty as a whole. Of course, if you find that the appliance is strange to you or that, after examining the records (which should be done before seeing the patient), you see that the case has gone way beyond its expected treatment time, you are doing neither party a favor by accepting the case.

Once you decide to accept the patient, however, you also accept all responsibility for future sequelae—in other words, you "own" the case. Miller recommends that you treat the transfer exam the same as any other new patient. Unless the referring orthodontist forwards exit records, you should take, as a minimum, facial and intraoral photos and a panorex (to check for root resorption and parallelism and bone loss) and enter into a contractual agreement. If there are only a few months of treatment remaining, a simple per-visit charge plus a fee for appliance removal, retainers, and records is made. If, on the other hand, a longer effort is expected, a comprehensive fee should be assessed. In any case, making negative comments that might reflect on the competency of the transferring orthodontist is a no-no![4]

Removal of braces placed elsewhere. When an orthodontist removes braces placed by another, he or she becomes part of the chain of treatment, which has legal implications should a malpractice suit be filed. If it is an emergency situation, the AAO member is obligated by the AAO Code of Ethics to help the patient as needed. In such case, the patient or parent should sign a waiver stating that the orthodontist is engaged solely for the purpose of removing the braces.

Although state laws differ, in many instances the process of removing braces confers the duty to diagnose upon the doctor, so that if the orthodontist fails to recognize a potential issue that a dentist would ordinarily be expected to recognize, the orthodontist may be held liable should the issue later develop into a full-blown malpractice case. Orthodontists who use CBCT imaging should have their scans read by a qualified dental radiologist.

Patient Who Attempts to Direct Treatment

Pleasing the patient—or parent—should never involve any compromise of the orthodontist's professional judgment. As orthodontists, we want to please our patients. However, there is a fine line between pleasing the patient and agreeing to a treatment that may not correct the problem in our opinion.

The initial treatment contract should include a clause stating that the orthodontist has designed a treatment plan that the patient or parent has reviewed and now accepts the doctor's judgment. Then, any challenge to the treatment plan may constitute a breach of contract.

Your best defense against possible litigation is quality diagnostic records and a written treatment plan explaining the proposed treatment, possible options, and your explanation of the alternatives and risks involved. When someone has unrealistic expectations of treatment and does not seem amenable to adjusting these expectations during the consultation, the orthodontist should think carefully about accepting that person as a patient. AAO members may download a copy of the supplemental informed consent form, "Patient declines treatment," which will help prevent you from being accused of not informing the patient.[5]

Verbal Abuse

What should you do if a patient's anger is frightening the staff or interfering with proper treatment procedures? Before such a situation occurs, your treatment contract should stipulate that patient behavior such as verbal abuse of the office staff may result in termination of treatment. Despite your best efforts to assuage the angry patient or parent, the following steps can be taken:

- ➢ If the behavior is physically aggressive or appears to be headed that way, the police should be contacted immediately. They will advise you of the steps to be taken—possibly the filing of a restraining order.
- ➢ When the doctor's attempts to assuage the disrupter have failed, the doctor-patient relationship has deteriorated to the point where effective treatment can no longer be accomplished, then, if not contraindicated, treatment should be terminated.
- ➢ Some orthodontists are reluctant to terminate a patient for fear of reprisal in the form of regulatory or malpractice complaints. In a practical sense, if such abuse occurs, it is probably inevitable that a malpractice allegation will be forthcoming.
- ➢ Finally, report a potential claim to your professional liability insurance company. They will not only open a claim file, but they also assist you in dealing with the situation.

> ➤ Depending on how far the situation has progressed, you may wish to contact your attorney or state dental board.[6]

Terminating a Patient

If termination has been decided upon, then you should proceed as follows, in writing:

1. Inform the patient (or guardian) as to the status and condition of treatment.
2. Recommend that they promptly secure the services of another orthodontist, offer to assist them in so doing, and explain that serious consequences could result if treatment is not immediately undertaken.
3. Select a definite date upon which the relationship will be terminated, which should be enough to secure other orthodontic care, but should be not less than 30 days after oral notice of intent to terminate.
4. Explain that you will be available on an emergency basis during the period between the oral notice and the effective date of termination (ie, the 30-day period).
5. Offer to make copies of the patient's records upon receiving proper request.
6. In the case wherein termination is based on the patient's failure to keep appointments, the letter should state, in addition to the above items, that you are confirming the patient's termination of the relationship by virtue of failing to appear for appointments (as opposed to your termination). This letter should be mailed by certified mail, return receipt requested.

ADULT TREATMENT

Dr David R. Musich, author and educator, offers these caveats in treating adults.

Treatment Goals

may have to differ from the ideal, especially if esthetics takes priority.

Misdiagnosis

can occur if these problems are overlooked:

> Existing periodontal disease, including the effects of smoking
> Root resorption
> TMD might be missed if a functional exam is not given
> Transverse deficiency. This can be overlooked if an anteroposterior cephalogram is not taken. Many cases should be skeletally expanded with surgically assisted RME (SARME) based on the principle of distraction osteogenesis.

Treatment Planning

requires interdisciplinary treatment 70% of the time. Do not accelerate aging.

Mechanotherapy

New distraction techniques and mini-implant anchorage are available to broaden our capabilities.

The six major reasons for retreatment:

> Undiagnosed maxillary transverse skeletal deficiency
> Treatment requiring surgery (42% of retreatment problems)
> Unstable (or recrowding) of mandibular incisors (25%)
> Crowding of maxillary centrals and laterals (21%)
> Labioversion of mandibular incisors from an accidentally activated portion of a fixed retainer
> Poor patient compliance.[7]

OTHER RISKS

Property and liability risks

Reputation. As noted under Transfer Cases, it is inappropriate to criticize the work of others. Doing so can be costly. Reputational harm claims are the most expensive claims small business owners (orthodontists included) face, with an average cost of $50,000. What you should do:

> Avoid criticizing competitors in your patients' presence.
> Refrain from posting patient photos online without their permission.
> Avoid posting anything created by others without their consent.

Motor vehicle accidents. If your employee uses an automobile for office business (picking up supplies, going to the bank), you are liable in case of an accident. What you should do:

> Screen the staff person's driving record before sending him or her on an errand.
> Avoid calling or texting them while they are on the road.

Fire. Do not attempt to save money by neglecting or postponing office upgrades. Reducing or eliminating the risk of fire could save you from an average $35,000 claim. What you should do:

> Routinely check sprinkler systems, fire extinguishers, and other safety equipment.
> Keep seldom-used equipment unplugged.
> Do not overload electrical outlets; be sure to periodically check electrical cords for damage.
> Do not place papers or other combustibles near heat-producing equipment such as computers, printers, coffeemakers, or microwaves.

Personal injury. If a patient slips on a puddle of sterilizing fluid and injures her knee, you could be held for big damages. In the winter, slipping on the ice outside your office could trigger a lawsuit if you are the property owner. What you should do:

> Keep outside areas in good repair and clear of snow, ice, and anything slippery.
> Be sure walkways and stairways are well-illuminated.
> Use signs to alert visitors of a wet floor.

Consider the possibility of wind and hail damage and take appropriate steps to minimize it.

Despite all your precautions, a business owner's insurance policy will protect you against the unforeseen.[8] AAO legal counsel Kevin Dillard offers these additional caveats:

Gifts to Referring Doctors

"Even a $10 gift card for the coffee house next to the referring doctor's office is likely to be a problem if you send one for every patient that practice sends to you. Although state regulations may differ, a basket of fruit or flowers at the end of the year will often be within legal guidelines."

Pro Bono Treatment for Employees

If a staff member, or his or her child, is under treatment, but leaves the practice unexpectedly, the orthodontist is still obligated to complete the treatment and has no legal basis to initiate a fee for it.

Avoiding Antitrust Pitfalls

If two or more orthodontists collude on fees, it would be a violation of the Sherman Antitrust Act because it is unlawful to engage in agreements that restrict trade. Organizing a boycott against a supplier whose prices seem out of line by a number of orthodontists would also be a clear violation of the statute.[9]

If a Patient Requests a Refund

Considering refunding all or part of a fee to prevent malpractice allegations is a business decision. It may be an appropriate way to resolve the issue. In other words, use a fee refund as a business decision and a PR tool. In most cases, it is not an admission of liability. Emphasize to the patient or parent that you believe your treatment was appropriate and within the standard of care. Tell them that, if they are willing to sign a release, you are willing to offer the refund to facilitate customer satisfaction, and be sure the release is signed before disseminating the money. The release should state that the refund is not an admission of liability and that the patient will not bring civil action against the doctor. It's a small price to pay to avoid having to defend yourself in a formal malpractice action. What's more, a fee refund is not reportable to the National Practitioner Data Bank.[10,11]

PRACTICING DEFENSIVELY

In our increasingly litigious society, which raises patients' expectations and, at the same time, reduces tolerance for doctors' errors, it behooves us to implement simple risk management strategies for the purpose of minimizing the possibility of legal action and at the same time ensuring a high level of treatment. Drs Ahmad Abdelkarim and Laurance Jerrold, writing in the August 2015 *AJO-DO*, offer these strategies, among others:

> ➤ Take excellent quality and comprehensive records, before, during, and after treatment.
> ➤ Meticulously clear every patient for orthodontic treatment.
> ➤ Obtain the appropriate informed consent from each patient.
> ➤ Do not promise or guarantee anything, and outline the limitations of treatment.
> ➤ Offer and discuss the orthognathic surgery option if it is viable.
> ➤ Document existing TMD, and do not manage it with orthodontic therapy alone.
> ➤ Scrupulously monitor patient's oral hygiene.
> ➤ Avoid invasive procedures when possible.
> ➤ Use protective eyewear on patients during every appointment.
> ➤ Discuss the importance and limitations of retention.[12]

CHAPTER XV

Orthodontic Education and Trends

THE "CRISIS" OF 2001

Dr Larry W. White, educator and editor of the *JCO*, described the state of orthodontic education in 2001. He called the situation a "crisis." At least 10 chairs of orthodontic programs lay vacant. Approximately 100 full-time positions in orthodontic departments remained unfilled.

Educational institutions complained that they couldn't compete for personnel because of low salaries, yet many of the schools severely limited what their faculty could earn on the outside. More and more schools were insisting that chairs come with PhDs. Another barrier was that schools gave tenure only to those who published in highly ranked journals. Not a single orthodontic journal worldwide was ranked in the upper first or second tiers of publication, meaning that orthodontic PhDs would need to publish in fields completely outside orthodontics.

Many potential professors simply decided that they couldn't afford to teach full-time with all the institutional restrictions on their earning power. A second feature of this crisis was the economics of running orthodontic departments. There seemed to be a schoolwide dependence on ortho departments. Deans had to scramble to find funds wherever they existed.

Of the 300 orthodontic residents who graduated each year, 100 of them were foreign-born, and they returned to their homelands, leaving only 200 to replace the 300–500 orthodontists who then retired each year. Although orthodontists may think a shortage of competition is a good thing, they should not expect the public or the federal and state governments to feel the same way.

Another problem was that more universities had extended their orthodontic curricula to 3 years, but a study showed that there were no measurable differences in 2-year graduates and those of 3 years. So we may be doing the residents and the public a disservice by insisting on a third year.[1]

THE "CRISIS" OF 2016

Dr David L. Turpin, faculty member at the University of Washington and editor emeritus of the *AJO-DO*, in an e-mail to the author on March 3, 2016, opined that the "crisis" now has more to do with student debt than with vacancies in teaching positions. He has in mind debts of $300,000 to $600,000. Some neophyte orthodontists must work (in most cases, for others) as many as 6 days a week to survive. Several private orthodontic schools are opening, with very high tuitions, just contributing to the problem. Not that established schools are cheap: Annual tuition at the University of the Pacific Arthur A. Dugoni School of Dentistry is $104,585 for the ortho program. Even so, the department receives 200 applications for the coveted eight spots per class.

The problem of unfilled department heads has eased, but many chairpersons must still fight to get enough salaried faculty spots. And for many of these faculty, research grants—which would help pay their salaries—are hard to come by. Contrary to what White said, Turpin claims that most dental schools provide opportunities for faculty members to practice 1 day a week—some without a state license.

Most foreign students want to stay and practice or teach, but their governments require many of them to return to their native countries. If and when their school visas expire, the US government is only too glad to see them leave.

Turpin agrees that there is increased pressure for all researchers and some educators to "publish or perish" and that about half the orthodontic research findings are published in nonorthodontic journals because of their higher impact factor (the average number of citations received per paper published in that journal during the two preceding years). He winds up his assessment by saying that "if we have a problem in the world of publication it is that we have too many journals often eager to publish anything."

PREDICTING ORTHODONTIC NEED

Can we predict how many people will be seeking orthodontic treatment at a particular time in the future so that the demand can be balanced by the output of graduating practitioners? Turpin, writing in the February 2010 *AJO-DO*, pointed out the difficulties of trying to divine "things to come."

It is difficult to calculate unmet need based on the underlying populations because there might be financial and psychosocial reasons for not seeking professional care. "Considering only unmet need without factoring in the roles of economic, social, and cultural factors," according to L. Jackson Brown, consultant to the AAO, "can lead to large miscalculations of the amount of orthodontic care that will actually be used. . . ." Most orthodontists believe that an additional 30% in new patient starts per week would not jeopardize quality of care. The additional workload could be accomplished by

- ➢ altering the appointment schedule (41.9%)
- ➢ becoming more efficient personally (39%)
- ➢ increasing staff (37%)

> ➢ working more hours (20.9%)
> ➢ increasing staff hours (15%)
> ➢ increasing number of orthodontists.

An increasing number of young adults have chosen to have orthodontic services; however, the percentage of individuals in that age category who actually get strapped up (or "Invisaligned") is relatively small compared with that of teenagers, declining after age 35.

Factors that positively influence demand include population, prevalence of malocclusion, educational levels, income, and prepayment coverage, but health history, ethnicity, sex, and age also affect demand. The potential market for orthodontic services for adults in the United States is determined by the following fundamental factors:

> ➢ size of the population between ages 13 and 21
> ➢ size of the young adult population between 22 and 45
> ➢ extent and severity of malocclusion
> ➢ demand for orthodontic services
> ➢ degree to which orthodontic services have been provided
> to teenagers before they become young adults.

From 1998 to 2006, visits to orthodontic offices generally followed the ups and downs of the overall US economy: It declined during the economic contraction that began in 2001, then turned up in 2004. Over 90% of all visits for full-mouth orthodontic procedures were to specialists. During the last period of economic tough times, GPs still focused on other procedures and left orthodontics to the orthodontists. There have been declines in both gross billings and net income since the third quarter of 2008. The numbers of orthodontists are projected to grow more rapidly during the coming decades relative to the subpopulations most likely to seek care.[2]

RECAP OF RECENT HISTORY

The years since the closing of the 20th century have been driven by the crucial issues in orthodontic education, public awareness, economic fluctuations, professional defensiveness, practice commercialization, outside control, technology, and an increasing reliance on the computer. Eric Curtis, in his book, *Orthodontics at 2000*, sums up the final decades as they pertained to organized orthodontics:

The 1980s

Near the end of the 1980s, the AAO called the proposed OSHA regulations requiring extensive infection control procedures "redundant and overbroad." It did support mandatory hepatitis-B vaccination for all health care workers, as well as disinfection of touch or splash surfaces, proper waste disposal, use of gloves and masks, sterilization or disinfection of all instruments, but opposed mandatory fluid-resistant clothing, surgical caps or hoods, and fluid-proof shoe covers in orthodontic offices.

The 1990s

The AAO supported the government directive that employers of dental health care personnel must offer the hepatitis-B vaccination series at no cost to employees. In marketing, the AAO's national public relations and advertising campaign featured computer imaging. Magazine ads appeared in *Mademoiselle Family Circle* in 1990 featuring a new computer-generated smile. There were continued efforts to promote the inclusion of orthodontic benefits in dental insurance policies.

In 1991, the AAO gave needed attention to orthodontic education, as T.M. Graber outlined 12 situations that must be addressed. The main points were the dearth of qualified teachers, waning federal funds for biomedical research, dental school closings, and public health trivialization of orthodontics.

The 1990s could be called the "regulatory decade." The National Practitioner Data Bank began operations in 1990. Infection control and office safety topped the list of practical problems to solve. The time had come to take more formal and strategic actions; for the first time, orthodontists became seriously involved in the political process. AAO members were asked to back the following:

> ➢ Mandatory drug testing of health care providers is not recommended by the Centers for Disease Control.
> ➢ All patients should be required, as part of the patient health history, to confidentially disclose their HIV and HBV status.
> ➢ The House and Senate should hold hearings and receive input from all interested parties before passing any definitive health care legislation.

In 1994, *orthodontics* became *orthodontics and dentofacial orthopedics*, as suggested by Tod Dewel in 1976, as its journal adopted a new name: *American Journal of Orthodontics and Dentofacial Orthopedics*. AAO president Clifford Marks told the House of Delegates in 1995 that "managed care is a euphemism for managed costs or perhaps, even more realistically, managing the caregiver."

Since the 1970s, the AAO had employed an in-house attorney. In 1995, it was the only dental specialty with a full-time legal counsel on staff. By '99, member services included annual sessions, insurance plans, library, placement services, government relations, conferences and seminars, practice administration, public relations, Concept Direct Reimbursement, legal counsel, media relations, brochures, marketing, videos, and risk management. The AAO was determined to take care of its own.[3]

The 2000s

Evidence-based orthodontics. Although evidence-based practice had gained acceptance in medicine as early as 1980 and was first defined in 1996, it was not until the opening of the 21st century that it had found its way into orthodontics. Dr Greg J. Huang, now orthodontic department head at the University of Washington, was one of its chief proponents. He recently stated that "evidence-based dentistry (EBD) provides a framework from which to objectively evaluate our literature." In his opinion, "knowing how to employ evidence-based methods is an invaluable skill that all practitioners should master."[4]

According to the ADA, EBD is based on three elements: the clinician's education and experience, the scientific literature, and the patient's values, preferences, and unique condition. And the literature must be evaluated by systematically examining many studies to determine the best approach.[5] Only then is the dentist prepared to proceed with treatment. The purpose of EBD is to "close the gap between what is known and what is practiced." What this means to the orthodontist is he or she must now have a greater understanding of complex research designs and statistics to practice effectively in today's demanding environment.[5]

Practice-based research network. In an effort to spur research and, at the same time, get the rank and file involved—even indirectly—in research, the National Institute of Dental and Craniofacial Research (NIDCR) in 2005 created a 7-year grant to develop regional networks of dental practices that would participate in coordinated prospective research projects. Thus was born the National Dental Practice-Based Research Network (NDPBRN). Its purposes are (1) to serve as an investigative partnership of practicing dentists and academic scientists, (2) to allow practitioners to propose or participate in research studies that address day-to-day issues in oral health care, and (3) to expand the dental profession's evidence base and further refine dental care.[6]

The AAO-PBRN has been instrumental in moving several orthodontic studies forward, including studies on adult anterior open bite, Class II, and root resorption.[7] To enroll, go to *http://www.nationaldentalpbrn.org*

How are we doing? Eugene L. Gottlieb, founder and editor of *JCO*, had these thoughts about the state of the specialty in 2007: Bracket-bonding was the most important technical advantage that he had seen. Self-ligating brackets eliminated the need for bracket ties. Noncompliance appliances, though effective, needed close attention to anchorage considerations, and functional appliances were still subject to debate. He also questioned the one-appointment consult as to whether orthodontists could make a thorough diagnosis.

From1981, when only 3% of orthodontic offices in the United States had a computer, to 2007, it was now a near-universal presence. The computer's unique capacity to store, analyze, and retrieve data has made it indispensable to practice management. In the past, when orthodontists were asked what they liked least about practice, the answer was "management." Gottlieb thought this was odd because that is exactly what they were doing.[8]

Orthodontists were not immune to the Great Recession of 2007–09:

> Seventy-five percent of practitioners experienced production declines.

> The sharp decline reduced demand for almost all dental services.

> Many prospective patients either began to shop around for lower fees or postpone treatment altogether.

> Some insurance companies started lowering reimbursements.

> With economies of scale on their side, corporate dental centers competed with solo orthodontic practices by offering lower fees and accepting more insurance.

> Unable to meet their retirement goals, many older orthodontists continued working, further increasing competition.

Women orthodontists. In 2008, the *JCO* reported that, over the past 6 years, the median age and the percentage of female orthodontists had increased 266.7% from the 1990 figure to 14.7% of the total. The following year saw the election of Dr Lili Horton as the first woman president of an AAO component society (PCSO). In 2013, Dr Gayle Glenn ascended to the presidency of the AAO itself.[9] Two years later, two other firsts occurred: The Edward H. Angle Society of Orthodontists announced the election of Valmy P. Kulbersh as its first female president, and, for the first time in history, the class entering the orthodontic program at the USC Herman Ostrow School of Dentistry was all female![10] These events were a far cry from the early days of the specialty when even being a woman orthodontist was a rarity. In 1932, for example, only 2 1/2% of US orthodontists were women. For a more complete list of women's firsts, see Table VII.

Table VII

Table VII. Firsts for Women Orthodontists

NAME	MILESTONE	DATE
Gertrude Locke	First woman to be a founding member of the ASO	1901
Anna H. Angle	First woman orthodontist to be ASO secretary; first to coedit *Angle Orthodontist*	1902; 1931
Guilhermena P. Mendell	First woman to graduate from Angle School; first to instruct there	1902
Jane G. Bunker	First woman orthodontist to be founding member of the European Orthodontic Society	1907
Josephine Abelson	First woman orthodontist to direct Dewey School Clinic	
Frances Genette Harbour	First woman orthodontist to practice in Los Angeles; first to be founding member of PCSO	1911; 1913
Elizabeth P. Richardson	First woman to head a university orthodontic dept.	1915
A. Florence Lilley	First woman orthodontist in Chicago	1919
Emily Hicks	First woman member of the Southwestern Society of Orthodontists	

Helen A. Gough	First daughter of an orthodontist (Frank A. Gough) to limit her practice and first woman orthodontist in Brooklyn	1924
Alice C. Kinninger	First woman to teach orthodontics at USC	1928
Eda B. Schlencker	First woman orthodontist to be ABO certified	1933
Carlotta A. Hawley	First woman to be accepted for graduate orthodontic training at Howard Dental School; first woman president of the Washington-Baltimore Society of Orthodontists	1938
Ruth Carter	First female and first black to be admitted to St Louis University orthodontic program	Ca. 1954
Augusta Dawson	First woman to be featured in *PCSO Bulletin*'s "Portrait of a Professional"	1989
Lili Horton	First woman president of a component society (PCSO)	2009
Gayle Glenn	First woman president of the AAO	2013
Valmy P. Kulbersh	First woman president of the Angle Society	2015

In other findings from the *JCO* survey, nearly half of all respondents were over the $1million mark in gross income. The most noteworthy finding was the rapid growth in routine usage of digital records. Digital cameras were now being used almost exclusively. The most commonly used analyses remained the Tweed, Downs, Steiner, Ricketts, and McNamara. Roth remained the most popular, standardized arch form.[11]

From 1982 to 2008, there was a 99% increase in the number of teenage orthodontic cases started by US orthodontists. By comparison, there was only a 15% increase in the teenage (12–17-year) population. During that same period, the number of adults who sought orthodontic treatment increased by 24%, yet the increase in adult population (age 18 and over) was 29.8%![12]

In terms of removable or functional appliances, more orthodontists were routinely using the Distal Jet, Class II Corrector, Forsus, banded Herbst, Invisalign, and MARA, according to the 2008 *JCO* survey. As far as skeletal anchorage was concerned, not more than 16% used miniscrews.[11]

The 2010s

As the economy was climbing out of the recession in 2010, the *McGill Advisory* reported that there were four options available for graduating residents: associateship, partnership, buyout, or start-up. Starting from scratch was the least viable. Costs—without buying a building—were between $300,000 and $500,000. It was more difficult to obtain financing than in the past. Then there was increased competition and the downturn in the marketplace. For these reasons, associateships were becoming increasingly difficult to find. The average practice was down between 10% and 20% for 2009 vs '08.

Another trend was the declining rate of treatment acceptance. Orthodontists were also advised to evaluate staffing. Most offices were overstaffed, the *Advisory* said. A guideline: one staff member for every $200,000 in collections.[13]

In 2012, there were approximately 136,000 GPs in the United States, according to the *Dental Tribune*. The largest specialty group, with a force of about 9,500, was orthodontists. Of the 65 graduate orthodontic programs in the country, the total resident enrollment at any given time was about 975, with about 360 graduating each year. Program length varied between 24 and 36 months. In the previous decade, the number of programs had substantially increased, triggering an 18% rise in the number of orthodontists coming out per year compared with the previous decade. There were also an increasing number of dental clinics and corporate-managed dental offices adding orthodontics to their menu.[14]

From *JCO's* 2013 survey, it was determined that the best practice-building methods were, in decreasing order,

> ➢ being on time for appointments
> ➢ finishing cases on time
> ➢ improving case presentation
> ➢ not charging for initial visit
> ➢ changing practice location
> ➢ treating adult patients

> improving staff management
> enhancing patient education[15]

Continuing the trend, AAO members in 2014 saw the following:

> an increase in both collections and net practice income for nearly 60%
> 46% of their patients being referred by dentists
> their average new-patient start figure go to 248 annually
> more than one fourth of their patients were adults.[16]

In a 2014 article in the *Orthodontic Cyberjournal*, Jerry Clark wrote that we were becoming more efficient because of direct bonded appliances; custom-fit bands; ceramic bonded brackets; space-age, heat-sensitive, Ni-Ti wires; polymeric ligatures; advances in surgery; new treatment techniques; computer-aided diagnosis and treatment planning; and expanded utilization of auxiliaries, all aimed to reduce chair time.[17]

Two years later, another piece of good news was announced by the National Center for Health Statistics and the Centers for Disease Control and Prevention: 50% of American women in the age bracket 15 to 44 said that they expect to have a child, an increase of 46% over the 2002 figure.[18]

CHAPTER XVI

SUMMATION OF PART TWO

The forces besetting orthodontics in the latter half of the 20th century continued into the 21st century. By this time, members of the profession had begun taking these forces in their stride, even though some, especially government control, the declining birth rate, consumerism, and technology had gained momentum. In the words of practice consultant Chris Bentson, "Running a successful practice is [becoming] increasingly complex and the path leading to financial success seems steeper than past years."[19]

Specific Conclusions

A. Economic
1. The Great Recession of 2007–09 affected orthodontists more than any other dental specialty.
2. The cost of dental and orthodontic education grew out of reach of many aspirants.
3. Competition has increased from both the output of new graduates and openings of new MSOs.
4. Increased student indebtedness has prevented most orthodontic residents from opening their own offices after graduating.
5. The delay in older practitioners' retirement has caused the number of available associateships to drop.

B. Government control
1. Consumerism and complaints have resulted in new government regulations, both at the federal and state levels, particularly with respect to OSHA and infection control.
2. The computer, with its social media and ability to instantly expose wrongdoing—real or perceived—has accelerated regulatory control.

C. The birthrate continues to decline. It is now at its lowest ebb.

D. Corporate orthodontics
1. The increasing difficulty of starting a new orthodontic practice has made corporate orthodontics more attractive to new graduates.
2. More corporate-managed dental offices are offering orthodontic services.

3. Lower fees proffered by MSOs have created downward pressure on those of private offices.

E. Interdental relationships
1. There has been a decrease in GP and specialty referrals.

F. Orthodontic education
1. New dental schools, with their attendant potential for turning out additional orthodontists, continue to open.
2. Between 2000 and 2012, the number of graduating orthodontic residents increased approximately 20%, yet the increase in US population was only 11%.
3. Most residents feel that, in their training programs, not enough attention is being paid to the management aspects of practice.
4. Competition for admission to orthodontic programs is still keen.
5. For those fortunate enough to gain admission, tuition has reached record proportions, burdening students with insurmountable debt.

G. Technology
1. The computer has had the greatest nonclinical impact on orthodontic practice.
2. The most important innovations wrought by computers are in the fields of record-keeping, appointments, imaging, treatment planning, use of the Web, and social media.
3. There was increased usage of Invisalign, self-ligating brackets, surgical adjuncts, indirect bonding, and bonded molar attachments and retainers.
4. The use of headgears and positioners declined.

H. Practice management
1. The orthodontist's role has changed from wire-bender to manager.
2. There has been an increase in the delegation of tasks to auxiliaries, such as case presentations and fee arrangements.
3. Staff sizes have consequently undergone a concomitant increase: The typical busy office now has a staff of seven full-time and two part-time employees.
4. There has been an increase in internal marketing programs.
5. Fee and payment arrangements are changing.
6. Insurance issues have multiplied.
7. The one-appointment consult has become more common.

I. Cosumerism/litigation
1. A Web presence has become a must for placing one's practice before the public.

2. This has elevated the patient from a "case" to a "consumer."

3. Consumerism has led to increased patient demands, government legislation, and practitioners' defensiveness.

OUTLOOK

Dr Duncan Y. Brown of Calgary, Canada, believes the golden age is not over: We are better prepared to understand the factors that contribute to patient satisfaction. We are better able to respond to patient needs. CBCT radiography, self-ligating brackets, advanced diagnosis and treatment concepts, TADs, and soft tissue lasers have contributed to contemporary orthodontic practice and improved the lives of our patients.[20]

What of the future?

David Turpin prognosticates that the orthodontic community will become more globalized. "Huge meetings are now being held throughout the world, with the most successful taking place in Southeast Asia and the Middle East." There are now more than 530 dental schools in India and 350 orthodontic programs. China has over 500 dental schools. The ortho residents at the Peking School of Dentistry are now taught exclusively in English. (E-mail to author, October 6, 2016.)

When forward-looking orthodontists talk about research, education, and board certification, they mention the word WFO (World Federation of Orthodontists) as often as AAO was mentioned 50 years ago. Thanks to the computer and air travel, the AAO is only one of WFO's 89 affiliates. Some of the 10,000-member organization's goals are to encourage and assist in the formation of national and regional certifying boards, promote orthodontic research, act as a co-organizer of the International Orthodontic Congress (held every 5 years), and encourage high orthodontic standards throughout the world.[21]

Students worldwide will be able to simultaneously attend interactive classes. Study models will be digital. 3-D printers will be used whenever physical models are needed. Technological advances will facilitate convenient custom-designed treatment. Information technology will bolster patient care by assisting work flow. Tooth-movement control systems will alert orthodontists whenever they divert from treatment goals. Patients, in turn, will interact more with the treatment.[22]

Dr Terry Sellke, educator and founder of *The Bottom Line*, sums up the outlook for orthodontics: The teen population will remain below 2004 numbers. Only Hispanic births are up. The supply of orthodontist graduates will remain ample. Fewer orthodontists are retiring. Some doctors will simply close their doors. Some will find a willing new graduate to buy their practices. Still others will sell to a corporate entity. As for managed care, what happened to medical doctors could happen to us: By 1984, the MDs had lost their independence forever, as managed care patients represented such a huge portion of their practices that they could no longer afford to "opt out."

Government intervention is here to stay. It will be setting the fees, determining the services to be rendered, and doling out care with a limited budget. We will merely be adding Obamacare to Social Security, Medicare, and Medicaid as governmentally run entitlement programs that our nation can no longer afford. As the cost of health care increases, businesses will look for ways to cut expenses. Dentistry may be a good place for them to begin. Indemnity programs will become a thing of the past. HMOs will deny care to those who need it. Orthodontics will be at the top of the list of services that will be dropped as a cost-containment measure. Sellke sees that as a boon to orthodontists who, free from third-party intrusion, can educate the public about the benefits and value of orthodontics and can convince patients that theirs is the practice to come to. The successful orthodontist will be the one who can differentiate his or her practice: consumers seek convenience and speed. It is not enough to say you are "better" or "faster." You must document it. You must have a Web site. Sellke treats all fully banded cases with SureSmile. He also uses AcceleDent to hasten tooth movement.[23] (See Chapter XII, Accelerated Tooth Movement.)

Despite these challenges, I think we're pretty well off. According to *The Atlantic's* 2013 survey of America's best-paying jobs, orthodontists have the fifth-highest-paying occupation. To be in the top four, you'd have to be a physician or surgeon.[24] At least we can go to sleep at night without worrying whether our patients will live or die.

The Bureau of Labor Statistics reported that, in May 2014, the mean annual income of orthodontists was $201,030. The mean hourly rate was $96.65. We were also ranked as No. 1 among the 100 best jobs, as well as No.1 in the best health care jobs.[25] In 2016, *US News and World Report* listed orthodontics as the No. 1 job in America.[26] As to whether we're still in the golden age, I don't think that argument will ever be settled because job satisfaction involves more than remuneration. Perhaps it should be called the age of gold.

REFERENCES FOR PART TWO

CHAPTER IX
1. Gottlieb EL, Nelson AH, Vogels DS III. 2001 *JCO* practice study, Part I: Trends. *J Clin Orthod.* 2001;35:623–631.
2. Klempner L. Wave goodbye to the good old days. *Orthod Products.* 2015;Feb.:24–25.
3. Waldman HB, Perlman SP, Schindel R. Update on the imbalanced distribution of orthodontists, 1995–2006. *Am J Orthod Dentofacial Orthop.* 2009;135:704–708.
4. J.Z. US women are having fewer babies than ever. *Time.* August 29, 2016. p. 21.
5. Ruse A. The cause of America's declining birthrate. Available at: http://www.Crisismagazine.com. Accessed October 18, 2014.
6. Galbreath RN, Hilgers KK, Silveira AM, Scheetz JP. Orthodontic treatment provided by general dentists who have achieved master's level in the Academy of General Dentistry. *Am J Orthod Dentofacial Orthop.* 2006;129:678–686.
7. Orthodontics and the general practitioner. *J Am Dent Assoc.* 2002;133:369–371.
8. Du Molin J. General dentist orthodontics: the war is on. http://the wealthydentist.com/author/twd_admin/. Accessed October 21, 2014.
9. DePaul R. Drive new patients to your practice using cosmetic orthodontics. *Dent Econ.* 2008;98:n.p. http://www.dentaleconomics.com/articles/print/volume-98/issue-12/features/focus-on/drive-new-patients-to-your-practice-using-cosmetic-orthodontics.html
10. Abei Y, Nelson S, Amberman D. Comparing orthodontic treatment outcome between orthodontists and general dentists with the ABO index. *Am J Orthod Dentofacial Orthop.* 2004;126:544–548.
11. Mascarenhas AK, Vig K, Joo B-H. Patients' satisfaction with their child's orthodontic care: a comparison of orthodontists and pediatric dentists. *Pediatr Dent.* 2005;27:451–456.
12. Oppenhuizen G. Management service organizations in orthodontics: a paradigm shift? *Am J Orthod Dentofacial Orthop.* 1997;112:345–347.
13. Dental management service organizations. http://www.mcgregorfirm.com/dental_mso.php. Accessed October 18, 2015.
14. Sfikas PM. Are MSOs and orthodontists partners? *J Am Dent Assoc.* 2006;137:536–537.
15. Hoffman J. [No title]. http://www.dental-tribune.com/articles/news. Accessed October 30, 2014.

16. Karkaria, U. A dream dissolved. *Florida Times-Union*. 2006. http://jacksonville.com/tu-online/stories/092406/. Accessed October 31, 2014.

17. The Roundtable: corporate orthodontics. *Orthod Products* Online. http://www.orthodonticproductsonline.com/2013/07/the-roundtable-corporate-orthodontics/. Accessed November 3, 2014.

18. What's it like doing corporate orthodontics? http://www:dentaltown.com. Accessed October 19, 2014.

19. Bunn BJ. Effects of management service organizations on traditional orthodontists. *Am J Orthod Dentofacial Orthop*. 2000;117:A1.

20. Clark JR. The management revolution. *Orthod Cyberjournal*. Accessed October 13, 2014.

CHAPTER X

1. Taking control of infection control. *Orthod Products*. 2015 (March);24–27.

2. Infection reminders for dental offices. *CDA Update*. 2016;28(7):11.

3. Harris T. "O(Oh) S(Shucks) H(Here) It is A(Again)." *PCSO Bull*. 2007;25:36–37.

4. Dentists must comply with new medical waste law. *CDA Update*. 2015;27(7):4.

5. Dentists cited for not having Cal/OSHA required plans. *CDA Update*. 2015;27(3);8.

6. OSHA updates eyewash station resource. *CDA Update*. 2015;27(9):6.

7. Cuny E. Hazard communications and hazardous waste regulations for dental offices. Available at: http://www.dentalcare.com/media/en-US/education/ce55/ce55.pdf. Accessed December 15, 2015.

8. Infection control Q-and-A. *CDA J*. 2016;44:135–138.

9. Uses and disclosures of patient health information: part I. *CDA J*. 2015;43:267–270.

10. Handle Social Security numbers and driver's licenses carefully. *CDA Update*. 2016;28(5):11–12.

11. New resource helps dentists become HIPAA-compliant.*CDA Update*. 2015;27(10):4.

12. Seven cyber liability questions for your practice. *The (AAO) Bull*. 2016;34:16–17.

13. ACA impact to vary from state to state. Retrieved October 10, 2014 from http://www.aaoinfo/org.news/201312/

14. Qualifying for medically necessary orthodontic treatment under the Affordable Care Act. *AAO Bull*. 2014;32:12–13.

15. Overview: the Federal Truth in Lending Act. *The (AAO) Bull*. 2015;33:14–18.

16. Ford DT. Are electronic health records the future of dental practice? *CDA J*. 2015;43:239-243.

17. Mostofi S, Hoffman AL. Legal considerations for electronic health records. *CDA J.* 2015;43:245–249.

18. Krauthammer C. Turning doctors into typists. *The Week.* 2015 (June 12):12.

19. Dental Board of California: continuing education requirements. Retrieved from cda.org/portals/0/pdfs/condensed_ce_n. February 10, 2015.

CHAPTER XI

1. Franklin E. Enamel damage during adhesive removal leads to big malpractice claims. *The (AAO) Bull.* 2015;33:24–25.

2. Maués CPR, do Nascimento RR, Vilella OV. Severe root resorption resulting from orthodontic treatment: prevalence and risk factors. *Dent Press J Orthod.* 2015;20(1): 52–58.

3. Wahl N. Orthodonics in 3 millennia. Chapter 13: The temporomandibular joint and orthognathic surgery. *Am J Orthod Dentofacial Orthop.* 2007;131:263–267.

4. Reynders RM. Orthodontics and temporomandibular disorders: A review of the literature (1966-1988). *Am J Orthod Dentofacial Orthop.* 1990;97:463-471.

5. Morrison K. The evolution of social media [infographic]. Retrieved August 27, 2016, from http://www.adweek.com/socialtimes/the-evolution-of-social-media-infographic/620911

6. Franklin E. Social media and malpractice. *The (AAO) Bull.* 2014;32:30-31.

7. Franklin E. Why do patients sue orthodontists? *The (AAO) Bull.* 2014;32:22–23.

8. Handle office accidents properly to prevent malpractice claims. Retrieved from https://www.aaoinfo.org/legal-advocacy/legal-issues/handle-office-accidents-properly-prevent-malpractice-claims. Retrieved May 25, 2015.

9. Franklin E. Kids, poor oral hygiene and malpractice claims. *The (AAO) Bull.* 2015;33:24–25.

10. Machen DE. Practice Management: Why are orthodontic lawsuits initiated . . . and why are they lost? *Orthotown Magazine.* 2010 (Apr);56–59.

11. Gottlieb EL. Don't rest on your laurels. *J Clin Orthod.* 1995;29:619–620.

12. Nelson G. Orthodontic practice in a time of economic stress. *PCSO Bull.* 2009 (fall);27:4–5.

13. Sellke T. The new economy reality check: where does that leave us? *Progressive Orthodontist Magazine.* Available at: https://www.aaoinfo.org/system/files/media/documents/Sellke%20--%20The%20Future%20of%20Orthodontics%3B%20The%20Next%20Ten%20Years.pdf Accessed August 13, 2015.

14. Diringer J, Phipps K, Carsel B. Critical trends affecting the future of dentistry: assessing the shifting landscape. Available at: http://www.ada.org/~/media/ADA/Member%20Center/FIles/Escan2013_Diringer_Full.ashx. Accessed September 11, 2015.

15. Nelson C. Consumerism in the dental industry—understanding the new dental consumer. Available at: http://sidekickmag.com/dental-practice-management/consumerism-in-the-dental-industry-understanding-the-new-dental-consume/[stet]. Accessed February 11, 2016.

16. How to file a complaint against an orthodontist. Available at: http://www.howtodothings.com/careers/how-to-file-a-complaint-against-an-orthodontist. Accessed November 5, 2015.

17. If you receive a patient complaint, summons, or regulatory body complaint: Available at: https://aaoic.com/aaoic-enews-spring-2014. Accessed November 8, 2015.

18. Oakley C. 3 people dish: surviving with massive student loan debt. Retrieved September 13, 2016, from: http://www.forbes.com/forbes/welcome/?/sites/learnvest/2013/06/06/3-people-dish-surviving-with-massive-student-loan-debt

19. Corbell T. 5 Solutions to ease the pain of your student loan debt. *The Biz Coach*. Retrieved September 13, 2016, from: http://www.bizcoachinfo.com/archives/13843

20. Arpino VJ. Dear alumni, colleagues and friends. Available at: http://textlab.io/doc/522813/orthodontic-alumni-newsletter-2013---university-of-illinois. Accessed November 13, 2015.

21. Overcash L. Residents' survey. *Orthod Products*. 2014. Available at: http://www.orthodonticproductsonline.com/2014/08/residents-survey/. Accessed January 15, 2015.

22. Caldwell M. 7 steps to help you pay off your student loans. Retrieved December 8, 2015 from: moneyfor20s.about.com/od/managingyourstudentloans

23. Pruzansky DP, Ellis B, Park JH. Influence of student-loan debt on orthodontic residents and recent graduates. *J Clin Orthod*. 2016;50:23–32.

24. Keim RG. The burden of student debt (editorial). *J Clin Orthod*. 2016;50:9–10.

25. Keim RG, Gottlieb EL, Nelson AH, Vogels, DS III. *JCO* survey of referring dentists. *J Clin Orthod*. 2004;38:219–223.

CHAPTER XII

1. McGuire MK, Scheyer ET, Gallerano RL. Temporary anchorage devices for tooth movement: a review and case reports. *J Periodontol*. 2006;77:1613–1624.

2. Choo H, Kim SH, Huang JC. TAD, a misnomer? *Am J Orthod Dentofacial Orthop*. 2009;136:145–146.

3. Piehler C. TADs usage survey: How and how often do orthodontists use temporary anchorage devices? *Orthod Products Online*. 2012. Available at: https://www.highbeam.com/doc/1G1-393875147.html. Accessed October 20, 2015. [https://en.wikipedia.org/wiki/distraction_osteogenesis]

4. Distraction osteogenesis. Wikipedia. Available at: https://en.wikipedia.org/wiki/Distraction_osteogenesis. Accessed December 5, 2015.

5. Wahl N. Orthodontics in 3 millennia. Chap. 14: Surgical adjuncts to orthodontics. *Am J Orthod Dentofacial Orthop*. 2007;131:561–565.

6. Kusy RP. Orthodontic biomaterials: from the past to the present. *Angle Orthod*. 2002;72:501–512.

7. Sachdeva RCL. Treatment time: SureSmile vs conventional. *Scientific innovation* 2012;13(1):72–85. Available at: http://www.osgb.com/pdfs/articles/clinical/Treatment%20Time%20-%20SureSmile%20vs%20Conventional.pdf. Accessed December 5, 2015.

8. Larson BE, Vaubel CJ, Grünheid T. Effect of computer-assisted orthodontic treatment technology to achieve predicted outcomes. *Angle Orthod*. 2013;83:557–562.

9. Saxe AK, Louie LJ, Mah J. World J Orthod 2010;11(1):16–22.

10. Weber DJ II. *Effectiveness and efficiency of customized versus conventional orthodontic system* [sic] [master's thesis]. Chapel Hill: University of North Carolina; 2011.

11. Werner A. Customized bracket and wire survey. *Orthod Products*. 2012. Available at: http://www.orthodonticproductsonline.com/2012/11/customized-bracket-and-wire-survey2/. Accessed February 10, 2016.

12. Rinchuse DJ, Miles PG. Self-ligating brackets: present and future. *Am J Orthod Dentofacial Orthop*. 2007;132:216–222.

13. Greenlee GM, et al. Systematic review of self-ligating brackets. *Am J Orthod Dentofacial Orthop*. 2010;137:726–727.

14. Alpan D. Dr. David Alpan discusses several technologies that deliver orthodontic treatment in less time. Retrieved January 15, 2017, from: https://www.orthopracticeus.com/ce-articles/review-accelerated-orthodontics

15. Andrade I Jr, Beatriz dos Santos Sousa A, Gonçalves da Silva G. New therapeutic modalities to modulate orthodontic tooth movement. *Dental Press J Orthod*. 2014;19(6):n.p.

16. Lee W, et al. Corticotomy-/osteotomy-assisted tooth movement microCTs differ. *J Dent Res*. 2008;87:861–867.

17. Alikhani M, Raptis M, Zoldan B, et al. Effect of the micro-osteoperforations on the rate of tooth movement. *Am J Orthod Dentofacial Orthop*. 2013;144(5):639–648.

18. Graber LW. Have beautiful, healthy teeth . . . at any age! *Bottom Line Health.* 2017(May);31(5):11–13.

19. Keski-Nisula K, et al. Orthodontic intervention in the early mixed dentition: a prospective, controlled study on the effects of the eruption guidance appliance. *Am J Orthod Dentofacial Orthop.* 2008;133:254–260.

20. Christensen GJ. Orthodontics and the general practitioner. *J Am Dent Assoc.* 2002;133:369–371.

21. Rinchuse Donald J, Rinchuse Daniel J. Orthodontics and the general practitioner. *J Am Dent Assoc.* 2002;133:1159–1160.

22. Ogodescu A, et al. The digital decade in interdisciplinary orthodontics. 2010. Available at: www.wseas.us/e-library/conferences/2010/TimisoaraP/.../ACC-18.pdf. Retrieved October 25, 2014.

23. Shastry S, Park JH. Evaluation of the use of digital study models in postgraduate orthodontic programs in the United States and Canada. *Angle Orthod.* 2014;84:62–67.

24. The American Board of Orthodontics. Digital model requirements. Available at: www.AmericanBoardOrtho.com. Retrieved June 6, 2016.

25. Park JH. The new digital era in orthodontics. *PCSO Bull Dig.* 2016;Summer:10–11.

26. Get tips on your cyber security for your practice. *CDA Update.* 2015;27:9, 14.

27. Top seven data breach considerations. *CDA J.* 2016;44:49, 52–53.

28. Protect credit card terminals in the office. *CDA Update.* 2016;28:8.

29. https://www.aaoinfo.org/news/2016/04/aao-cautions-public-new-diy-orthodontics-approach-gains-attention. Accessed November 8, 2016.

30. http://well.blogs.nytimes.com/2015/02/01/a-trip-to-the-mail-box-not-the-orthodontist/. Accessed November 8, 2016.

31. Behrents RG. Consumer alert on the use of elastics as "gap bands." *Am J Orthod Dentofacial Orthop.* 2014;146:271–272.

32. Keim RG. Keep it simple. *J Clin Orthod.* 2008;42:433–434.

CHAPTER XIII

1. Remington L. Keys to marketing your practice. *Clin Impressions.* 2006;15(1):n.p.

2. Guidelines for AAO members' use of AAO marketing and communication materials by constituents, components, groups, or individual members. Retrieved October 24, 2014, from https://www.aaoinfo.org/practice/marketing

3. Sichtermann L. Website analysis. *Orthod Products.* 2015;49:28–29.

4. August J. Using QR codes in your dental or orthodontic practice. 2011. Available at: http://my socialpractice.com/2011/08/qr-codes. Accessed April 11, 2016.

5. Levin RP. Achieving total orthodontic success in a down economy. *PCSO Bull.* 2010;28(Summer):40–43.

6. Behan J. The importance of office staff in marketing. *Clin Impressions.* 2008;12:32–35.

7. Husayni A. Management and marketing: a guide to ranking above your competition in Google search results. *J Clin Orthod.* 2011;45:637–639.

8. Newman B. Five social media tips for dental practices. *CDA Update.* 2015;27:8, 10.

9. Klempner L. Wave goodbye to the good old days. *Orthod Products.* 2015;49:24–25.

10. Huddleston C. How to save money on braces. *Kiplinger Online.* Available at: http://m.kiplinger.com/article/spending/T027-C011-S001-how-to-save-money-on-braces.html. Accessed October 23, 2015.

11. Hall JF, Sohn W, McNamara JA Jr. Why do dentists refer to specific Orthodontists? *Angle Orthodontist.* 2009;79:5–11.

12. Overcash L. More than 300 new doctors enter into the workforce yearly. *Orthod Products.* 2014;48:n.p.

13. Summers J. The consult. *Orthod Products.* 2015 (July):14.

14. Get license for waiting room movies at discounted rate. *CDA Update.* 2015;27:15.

15. Burris B. Focus on the business of orthodontics. 2014. Available at: https://www.google.com/#q=Burris+B.+Focus+on+the+business+of+orthodontics. Accessed June1, 2015.

16. Handle patient record requests the right way. *CDA Update.* 2016;28:1, 8.

17. The importance of contracts. *The (AAO) Bull.* 2014;32:10.

18. Bentson C. Practice Valuation 101. Retrieved from: http://www.bentsonclark.com/blog/tag/orthodontic-practice-valuations/. Accessed December 30, 2016.

19. Franklin E. Avoid malpractice claims early in your career with due diligence. *The (AAO) Bull.* 2016;34:26–27.

20. Strang, RHW. Highlights of 64 years in orthodontics. *Angle Orthod.* 1974,44.101–112.

21. Heying SS, et al. The success of orthodontic satellite practices. *Angle Orthod.* 2007;77:875–880.

22. California Dental Practice Act, 2013–2016. What your orthodontic assistant may and may not do. Available at: http://www.dbc.ca.gov/formspubs/pub_permitted_duties.pdf. Accessed January 18, 2015.

23. Sick leave law frequently asked questions. *CDA Update.* 2015;27:6.

24. 5 steps to take with leave of absence request. *CDA Update.* 2016;28:10.

25. New overtime laws released. *CDA Update.* 2016;28:10.

26. Understanding meal and rest break policies. *CDA Update.* 2016;28:10, 15.

27. Sick leave law compliance deadline. Available at: http://www.cda.org/news-events/sick-leave-law-compliance-deadline-approaching. Accessed May 19, 2015.

28. *The (AAO) Bull.* 2017;35(1):8–9.

29. What's your policy? *CDA Update.* 2017;29:1, 4.

30. Corbo M. How to handle disciplining dental staff. *CDA Update.* 2015;27:13.

31. Haeger, RS. Managing and marketing: establishing an optimal pricing strategy for your practice. *J Clin Orthod.* 2014;48:563-569.

32. Kravitz ND. Emergency protocol. *Orthod Products.* 2015 (April, May):50–53.

33. Bentson C, Copple D. Time to sell. *Orthod Products Online.* 2013. Available at: http://www.orthodonticproductsonline.com/2013/09/time-to-sell/. Accessed February 13, 2016.

CHAPTER XIV

1. Preface. In: Graber TM, Eliades T, Athanasiou AE, eds. *Risk Management in Orthodontics: Experts' Guide to Malpractice.* Chicago: Quintessence; 2004:vii–viii.

2. Graber TM. Risk management. Chap 12 in: *Risk Management in Orthodontics: Experts' Guide to Malpractice.* Chicago: Quintessence; 2004:185–186.

3. Collection policies and procedures. Retrieved October 24, 2014, from: https://www.aaoinfo.org/legal-advocacy/legal-issues/collection-policies-and-procedures

4. Miller SL. Transitioning transfers. *Orthod Products.* 2016 (June):24–28.

5. Varner R. Preventing a malpractice claim by a patient attempting to dictate treatment. *The (AAO) Bull.* 2015;33:24–25.

6. Franklin E. Difficult, angry patients/parents: minimizing malpractice exposure. Available at: https://www.aaoinfo.org/news/2013/09/difficult-angry-patientsparents-minimizing-malpractice-exposure. Accessed June 8, 2016.

7. Musich DR. Myths and misconceptions of adult diagnosis and treatment. Retrieved October 25, 2014, from: http://www.cdabo.org/lecturesdetail.asp?id=7

8. Pearl Insurance Co. Five property and liability claims that will destroy your bottom line. *The (AAO) Bull.* 2016 (Oct):24–25.

9. Salome N. Unforeseen patient issues can surface during orthodontic treatment. *The (AAO) Bull.* 2014;32:2–6.

10. Franklin E. Refund fees to prevent malpractice allegations. *The (AAO) Bull.* 2015;33:26–27.

11. Franklin E. Manage your reputation by managing patient dissatisfaction. *The (AAO) Bull.* 2015 (June);33:16–17.

12. Abdelkarim A, Jerrold L. Risk management strategies in orthodontics. Part 1: Clinical considerations. *Am J Orthod Dentofacial Orthop.* 2015;148:345–349.

CHAPTER XV

1. White LW. [No title]. *Orthod Cyberjournal.* 2001;June:n.p.

2. Turpin DL. Need and demand for orthodontic services: the final report. *Am J Orthod Dentofacial Orthop.* 2010;137:151–152.

3. Curtis EK. 1980–1989: the great communicators. In: *Orthodontics at 2000.* St Louis: American Association of Orthodontists; 2000:39–96.

4. Machado AW. An interview with Greg J. Huang. *Dent Press J Orthod.* 2015 Nov-Dec;20(6):32–36

5. Law SV, Chudasama DN, Rinchuse DJ. Evidence-based orthodontics. *Angle Orthod.* 2010;80:952–956

6. Kokich VG. Consider joining the orthodontic practice-based research network. *AJODO* 2013;144:323

7. [Announcement. No author, no title.] *AAO Web site.* https://www.aaoinfo.org/library-research/aao-practice-based-research-network. Accessed May 4, 2017.

8. Gottlieb EL, Keim RG. JCO interviews Dr. Eugene L. Gottlieb on 40 years of *JCO. J Clin Orthod.* 2007;41:489–500.

9. Pacheco A. Women in orthodontics—100 years to reach the top. 2012. *Yearbook* 2012 (formerly *World J Orthod*);13(1):n.p.

10. Thedailyfloss.com. Accessed October 22, 2016.

11. Keim RG, et al. 2008 JCO study of orthodontic diagnosis and treatment procedures. Part 1: results and trends. *J Clin Orthod.* 2008;42:625–640.

12. Evans DL. History of braces. Available at: http://www.davidevansdds.com/history_of_braces.php. Accessed March 18, 2016.

13. Dusek M, McGill J. How to weather the current economy as a younger orthodontist. *SAO Bull.* Retrieved October 25, 2014 from: http://www.mcgillhillgroup.com/pdf/SAO_2010_How_to_Weather_the_Current_Economy_as_a_Younger_Orthodontist_McGill.pdf

14. Benston AC. The business of private practice orthodontics in the United States. Retrieved October 19, 2014, from: https://www.google.com/#q=The+business+of+private+practice+orthodontics+in+the+United+States.+dental+tribune

15. Keim RG, et al. 2013 JCO orthodontic practice study. Part 1: trends. *J Clin Orthod.* 2013;47:661–671.

16. 2014 Economics Of Orthodontics Survey indicates practice management data mostly stable with growth in adult patient population. *The (AAO) Bull.* 2015;33:18.

17. Clark JR. The management revolution. *Orthod Cyberjournal.* Accessed October 13, 2014.

18. J.Z. More American women want to have children. *Time* 2016(Oct. 31):21.

19. Benston C. The business of private practice orthodontics in the United States. *Dent Tribune.* 2012;11–16.

20. Brown DY. Orthodontics' future, but bright. *Dent Tribune Canada.* 2011. Available at: http://www.dental-tribune.com/articles/specialities/orthodontics/6746_orthodontics_future_challenging_but_bright.html

21. About WFO. Available at: http://www.wfo.org/about-wfo/. Accessed May 4, 2017.

22. Faber J. Orthodontics of the future: from fiction to reality. *Dent Press J Orthod* (Brazil; online). 2010. Available at: http://www.scielo.br/scielo.php?pid=S2176-94512010000200001&script=sci_arttext&tlng=en. Accessed September 11, 2015.

23. Sellke T. The new economy reality check: where does this leave us? *Prog Orthod Mag.* 2003:14–17.

24. The best- and worst-paid jobs in America—in 1 very long chart. *The Atlantic.* Available at: http://www.theatlantic.com/business/archive/2014/06/the-best-and-worst-paid-jobs-in-americain-1-ludicrously-long-chart/373192/. Accessed March 3, 2016.

25. Bureau of Labor Statistics. 2014. Available at: www.bls.gov/oes/current/oes in.htm#27-0000

26. *US News & World Report* announces the 2016 best jobs. Accessed January 1, 2017, from http://www.usnews.com/info/blogs/press-room/2016/01/26/us-news-announces-the-2016-best-jobs

ABOUT THE AUTHOR

A native of Chicago and a West Point graduate, Norman Wahl was commissioned in the US Army Quartermaster Corps in 1946. After 3 years of service, he worked in the film studios, later producing two documentary films on the history of Los Angeles. He finally decided on a career in dentistry, specializing in orthodontics.

In addition to a BS degree from the US Military Academy, Dr Wahl has a DDS from the University of Illinois College of Dentistry, an MS in orthodontics from Northwestern University, and an MA in history from California State University at Northridge.

He has written for the military and lay presses as well as for dental publications, mostly on orthodontic history. He is the author of *Oral Signs and Symptoms, Wahl's Oral Histories, Who Was Who in Orthodontics with a Selected Bibliography of Orthodontic History*, and articles in the *American Journal of Orthodontics and Dentofacial Orthopedics* (including the 16-chapter series, "Orthodontics in 3 Millennia"), the *Angle Orthodontist, the Journal of Clinical Orthodontics, Dental Economics*, and the Pacific Coast Society of Orthodontists *Bulletin*. He has also taught orthodontic history at the UCLA College of Dentistry.

Dr Wahl lives with his wife, Betty, in Sequim, Washington, and divides his time between writing, freelance copyediting, and playing the piano for local retirement homes. *Golden Age* is an outgrowth of his master's thesis (CSUN, 1997). Having started his practice in 1963, he considers himself an eyewitness to the decline.

Index

CPSIA information can be obtained
at www.ICGtesting.com
Printed in the USA
LVHW081459190721
693089LV00015B/558

9 781506 904696